Y0-AWG-952

PAEDIATRIC HANDBOOK

Paediatric handbook

edited by
D C Geddis

*Senior Lecturer, Department of Paediatrics and Child Health,
University of Otago, New Zealand*

**William Heinemann Medical Books Limited
London**

William Heinemann Medical Books Limited
23 Bedford Square
London WC1B 3HH

First Heinemann edition 1982

Copyright © D C Geddis 1982

ISBN 0-433-11530-0

Computer Typesetting by Method Limited
8 The Broadway, Woodford Green, Essex, and
printed in Great Britain by Redwood Burn Limited
Trowbridge, Wiltshire.

Contents

Preface

This handbook provides information which is frequently
required about a number of paediatric conditions, particularly
those of an acute nature. It is not intended to replace adequate
discussion, consultation or reference to texts.

The book was compiled to provide answers to the most
common questions regarding treatment asked by practitioners
who have arrived at a diagnosis and are wondering just what to
do next. The guiding principle throughout has been to provide
for each condition simple, clear, practical, unambiguous
guidance which a relatively inexperienced practitioner can
follow – even at 3 a.m.

Members of each of the three paediatric departments of the
University of Otago have assisted in preparing this handbook
and contributions were also made by other hospital staff. I
wish to record the particular assistance of Dr C J Hewitt and
the clerical work of Miss K J Eunson.

D C GEDDIS
Dunedin 1982

University of Otago
Departments of Paediatrics and Child Health
Christchurch, Dunedin, Wellington

SIGGAARD-ANDERSEN ALIGNMENT NOMOGRAM

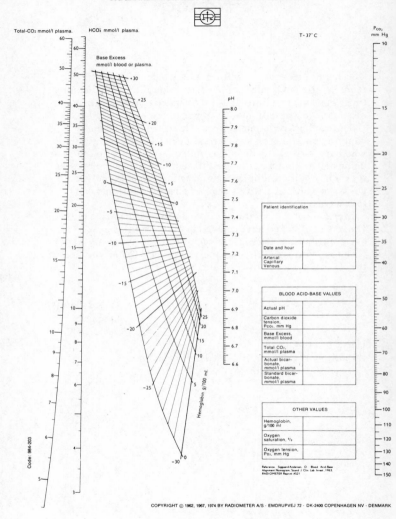

COPYRIGHT © 1962, 1967, 1974 BY RADIOMETER A/S · EMDRUPVEJ 72 · DK-2400 COPENHAGEN NV · DENMARK

Acid-Base Balance

Calculate base deficit from capillary or arterial blood gas values of pH and P_{CO_2} using Siggaard-Andersen Alignment Nomogram. Note that meq/l and mmol/l of base excess have the same numerical value.

Base deficit $\times$ 0.3 $\times$ weight in kg.
= No. of mmol of HCO_3^- needed
1 mmol = 1 ml of 8.4% $NaHCO_3$
Initially correct only half of calculated deficit and reassess.

Burns

Phases of Treatment

1. Ensure adequate airway
2. Adequate sedation
3. Assessment of extent of burn
4. Estimation of fluid replacement
5. Local treatment

Notes regarding transportation of burns patient

1. The most stable time is in the first 2 or 3 hours after the injury.
2. Remove burnt clothing. Children with burns have difficulty maintaining their body temperature so minimize heat loss through use of multiple dressings and sterile sheets.
3. If journey will take more than 2 hours insert an intravenous line.
4. Since ileus is a common and early complication insert a nasogastric tube.
5. Administer oxygen if carbon monoxide poisoning is suspected.
6. If inhalation injury is suspected consideration should be given to endotracheal incubation.

Airway

Check patency on arrival and periodically thereafter – especially in burns that have occurred indoors, when there is involvement of the face, or when prolonged exposure to smoke has occurred. In these situations restlessness may be on basis of hypoxia and not necessarily from discomfort of burn. Therefore assess patient carefully before administering sedation.

Sedation

Initially morphine 0.1-0.2mg/kg stat i.v.

Then morphine 0.1mg/kg i.m. as required.
Trimeprazine (Vallergan forte syrup) 3mg/kg 8-12 hrly.
Cold water or towels soaked in ice water is an effective way of controlling the pain from a burn. However, this should not be used for long periods, especially in burns of greater than 15%, since it can cause dramatic drops in body temperature.

Assessment of burn

1. Depth

Depth of Burn	Cause	Surface	Colour	Pain Sensation
Partial thickness (superficial)	Sun or minor flash	Dry, no blisters	Erythematous	Painful
Partial thickness (deep)	Flash or hot liquids	Blisters moist	Mottled red	Painful
Full thickness	Flare	Dry	Pearly white or charred	Little pain

2. Extent

| | Age in years | | | | |
	0	1	5	10	15
Head	18	15	13	11	8
Trunk	35	35	35	34	33
Arm	7	7	7	8	9
Thigh	12	14	15	16	18
Leg	8	9	10	11	12

% of surface area

Neck (2%), buttocks (5%), genitals (1%), hands (5%) and feet (7%) are not included in the above figures.
The area covered by the surface of an open hand is $1\frac{1}{2}\%$.
Note:
It is easy to over-estimate the burned surface area in a child, and this may cause problems from over-replacement of fluids.

Fluid Replacement

If burns are less than 10% and patient not vomiting give oral
fluids, especially milk. Watch urine output. More than 10%,
i.v. therapy as outlined below.

1. Weigh patient
2. Normal maintenance fluids:
    0.18% saline + 4% dextrose: (100 minus age in years × 3)
    ml/kg/day
3. Estimation of volume of replacement fluid
    % area burned × weight in kg × 2 = ml of fluids required in
    first 24 hours
    NB If % area burned is greater than 30% still only
    calculate as 30% to avoid overhydration.
4. Type of replacement fluid:
    In first 24 hours: Hartmann's solution (Ringer's lactate). No
    colloid added.
    In second 24 hours the replacement fluid should be equal
    parts Hartmann's solution and albumin.
    (The plasma deficit of colloid is estimated on the basis of
    0.5 ml albumin/kg body wt per 1% body surface burned).
    Note:
    With infants under 1 year of age use 0.18% saline + 4%
    dextrose in place of Hartmann's solution.
5. Rate of replacement:
    Divide fluid required/24 hours as calculated from 2 and 3
    above as follows:

Part I

First 8 hours: $\frac{1}{3}$ daily maintenance + half replacement volume
(as calculated from time of burn, not time of erecting i.v., e.g.
burn at 2pm, i.v. erected at 6pm, give Part I over 4 hours).

Part II

Next 16 hours: $\frac{2}{3}$ daily maintenance +, half replacement
volume.

Part III

Next 24 hours: Daily maintenance +, half replacement volume.

Part IV

Next 24 hours: (If necessary) Daily maintenance.

Urine Output

Hourly measurements. Observe carefully. Hourly rates are quite variable, so assess over period of 3 hours.
Oliguria is more commonly the result of inadequate fluid replacement than acute renal failure. However, urine volume of less than 0.5ml/kg/hour suggests renal failure. A test dose of mannitol may be given – 0.2g/kg i.v. over 5 mins should produce 6-10ml/kg of urine in 1-3 hours.

Normal Urine Output

Age	Vol. in ml/24 hours	ml/hour
1st-2nd day	30-60	1-3
3rd-10th day	100-300	4-12
10th-2 months	250-450	10-20
2 months-1 year	400-500	15-20
1-3 years	500-600	20-24
3-5 years	600-700	24-28
5-8 years	650-1000	30-34
8-14 years	800-1400	32-56

Local Treatment

Initially open exposure in room kept at 24-27°C.
(May require to be higher with extensive burns)

Procedure

1. All clothing removed.
2. Bed rest with all burned parts exposed freely to air if possible.
3. If this is not possible, burned part not exposed to air lies on sterile polyurethane.
4. All blisters excised.
5. Apply silver sulphadiazine cream b.d.
   Care should be taken over the use of this cream in children under 3 years of age as pyrexia may follow its application.
6. Splint areas of potential contracture.

Investigations

1. Hb, PCV and repeat alternate days.
2. If i.v. fluids – daily electrolytes and urea.
3. Plasma protein estimation – twice weekly.

Complications

1. Falling Hb may require top-up transfusion.
   Blood replacement: 1% blood volume per 1% burned.
   N.B. Blood volume = weight in kg × 75 in ml.
2. Infection. Daily swabs of burned area. Systemic, followed
   by oral penicillin if suspicious erythema develops around
   burn wound.
   Blood cultures as indicated clinically.
3. Ensure adequate calorie intake.
4. Monitor electrolytes since hyponatraemia is a common
   complication. Convulsions may occur in this situation.
5. Curling's ulcer – gastric erosions occur frequently with
   major burns. Give antacids as prophylactic measure.
6. Paralytic ileus – drip and suck.

Cardiovascular System

ACUTE HYPOXIC SPELL

Usually seen in patient with Tetralogy of Fallot. Spells not on basis of heart failure. Thought to be due to sudden, transient, increased right-to-left flow or to increased tissue demand for oxygen.

1. Pacify infant.
2. Place in knee-chest position.
3. Liberal oxygen.
4. Give morphine 0.2mg/kg stat i.m. (may repeat 4-6 hourly as necessary)
5. ± propanolol – either, 0.1mg/kg i.v. slowly to maximum of 5mg or, 0.2mg/kg i.m. stat.
6. May require $NaHCO_3$ – 5mmol/kg i.v. stat.

ACUTE PULMONARY OEDEMA

1. Place patient in sitting position.
2. Liberal oxygen. If necessary under positive pressure.
3. Morphine 0.2mg/kg s.c. or i.m. stat.
4. Frusemide (Lasix) 5mg/kg i.v. stat.
5. Digitalise (if this has not already been done). (*See* p.9).
   May also require:
   a. Aminophylline 5mg/kg i.v. slowly (over 15-30 mins).
   b. Application of tourniquets on three limbs in rotating fashion. Use blood pressure cuffs inflated to midway between systolic and diastolic pressure.
   c. Phlebotomy – 10ml/kg.

CARDIAC ARREST

1. Adequate airway
— bag and mask with O_2 at 6 1/min.
— intubate

age	diameter of tube
newborn	2.5mm
6/12 mo.	3.5mm
1 yr.	4.0mm
2 yrs.	5.0mm
4 yrs.	5.5mm
6 yrs.	6.0mm
8 yrs.	7.0mm
10 yrs.	7.5mm

2. External Cardiac Massage

Neonate — superimpose thumbs over middle of sternum, link fingers behind baby for support. Apply pressure with ball of lower thumb. 100/min

<5yrs. — Heel of hand just below midsternum. 80/min

5-10yrs. — Heel of hand over lower sternum. 60/min

Continue artificial respiration at a rate of 2 breaths/10 compressions (if only 1 attendant present) or 1 breath/5 compressions (if 2 attendants present)

3. ECG

(a) If asystole (majority of cardiac arrests in children due to this):
  (i) Adrenaline
    1:10 000 (0.1mg/ml)
    i.v. or intra-cardiac 0.01-0.05mg/kg (max 0.5mg)
  (ii) $CaCl_2$ 0.2ml/kg of 10% solution
    i.v. or intra-cardiac (min. 1ml; max. 10ml)
  (iii) $NaHCO_3$ 5mmol/kg i.v.
  (iv) Isoprenaline drip 0.5-1mg/250ml of 5% dextrose

Give as a continuous infusion. Titrate against heart
rate. Commence with 0.5-1ml/min
(b) If ventricular fibrillation:
  (i) defibrillation
     30-100watt/sec – infants
     100-300watt/sec – children
  (ii) NaHCO$_3$ 5mmol/kg i.v.

CARDIAC FAILURE

Consider heart failure in any infant presenting with
tachypnoea.

Assessment

1. History — pregnancy history – maternal infection with
             rubella; threatened miscarriage
          — feeding difficulties
          — cyanotic attacks
          — overtiredness and dyspnoea on feeding
          — precipitating factors e.g. chest infection
          — growth and development
2. Examination — weight (compare with previous records)
          — cyanosis
          — sweating
          — respiratory rate
          — peripheral pulses? absent femorals
          — liver enlargement and splenomegaly
          — murmurs and added sounds e.g. triple
            rhythm and ejection clicks
          — blood pressure. *NB* use correct cuff
          — A/P and lateral chest X-ray, ECG, Hb,
            WBC and diff.

Immediate Therapy

  1. Digitalise

    Always enquire of parents if child has received any
    digoxin in previous 48 hours.

| Digoxin – orally: | 0.08mg/kg/24 hours |
| i.m. or i.v.: | 0.06mg/kg/24 hours |

Give $\frac{1}{2}$ stat. In 12 hours give $\frac{1}{4}$ (after repeating ECG looking for signs of toxicity, e.g. prolongation of a-v conduction or premature ventricular contractions), and after a further 12 hours the remaining $\frac{1}{4}$.
Maintenance: 0.01-0.03mg/kg/day

Note:

In hospital check pulse before each dose.
Where a condition such as Fallot's Tetralogy is suspected, digitalis is relatively contraindicated.

2. Diuretic

Frusemide (Lasix) – 2mg/kg/stat/i.m.
Maintenance: 2-5mg/kg/day (in exceptional circumstances can increase to 10mg/kg/day)
If long-term therapy contemplated either:
Oral K – 1mmol/kg/day
or: spironolactone 2-5mg/kg/day in 2 divided doses
3. Liberal O_2 (humidified)
3. Nurse in head-up posture
5. Consider nasogastric tube feeding
6. Treat precipitating factors if possible e.g. chest infection, anaemia
7. May be some benefit in feeding with low sodium containing milk preparation
   e.g. breast milk
       some artificial preparations (*see* p.78)

Monitoring

Daily weight
Respiratory rate
Liver size
Initially urea and electrolytes alternate days
ECG
Chest X-ray } 1-2 weekly until stabilised

Note:

All children with congenital or acquired heart disease require penicillin before dental procedures e.g. extraction, scaling etc. (*see* p.19). All parents should be repeatedly reminded of this.

ECG

5 large squares = 1 sec.
10mm = 1 millivolt

1. Axis

(a) Determination:
Lead I: If R > S then axis to L. (0-90°)
   or (270-360°)
AVF: If R > S then axis inferior (0-180°)

(b) Normal:
Birth and neonatal period – R. ventricle dominant,
therefore axis > 90°. *NB* Prem. may have leftward axis
at birth which may persist for first couple of weeks.
Thereafter swings to right and subsequently behaves
normally. $\frac{2}{12} - \frac{3}{12}$ Axis usually starts to swing to L. and
is usually 0-90 by $\frac{6}{12}$ and should certainly be so by $\frac{12}{12}$.

2. P Wave

(a) Normally. Upright in I and II 0.08 sec. duration;
   < 2.5mm in ht..
May be of small amplitude and of shorter duration
during first $\frac{4}{52}$.

(b) R. atrial hypertrophy
P wave > 2.5mm
and peaked in   II V_1 V_4R

(c) L. atrial hypertrophy
Rare in children
> 0.12 sec. duration
± Neg. deflection towards end of P wave in V_1.

(d) If P inverted in I.
   (i) Check lead positions of L. and R. arms – may be
       transposed.
   (ii) Mirror image dextrocardia.
   (iii) Abnormal atrial focus (rare in children).

3. P-R Interval

(Onset of P to onset of QRS)
0.1-0.2 sec. Related to both heart rate and age of child.

Prolonged P-R interval:
(a) Acute myocarditis
(b) Drugs
        Digitalis
        Quinidine
        K^+
(c) Metabolic
        hypo- and hyperkalaemia
        Metabolic acidosis
        RDS
(d) Conduction abnormalities
        Ebstein's
        Endocardial fibroelastosis
        Endocardial cushion defect

Shortened P-R interval:
(a) Wolff Parkinson White Syndrome (+ delta waves)
(b) Muscular dystrophy
(c) Glycogenosis Type IIA (Pompe's Disease)

4. QRS

Duration gradually increases from birth.
Birth – 0.065 sec. – 0.08 adult
(a) Prolongation:
    (i) Complete a-v block
    (ii) RBBB : LBBB
    (iii) Hyperkalaemia
    (iv) Pompe's disease
(b) Shortening:
        Hyponatraemia

5. Q Wave

Children often have Q wave in I, II, III, AVF, V_5, V_6
Not pathological if < 5mm.

6. T Wave

The normal T wave is always +ve in I. Upright T waves in

the R chest leads are seen normally during the first week of life. After this they are definitely abnormal as in infants and children the T waves in V_1-V_3 should be inverted. Persistence of an upright T wave in V_1-V_3 may indicate RV strain. The age at which the T wave again becomes upright in the R chest leads is variable.

In contrast to signs of RV strain in infants and young children, the findings of inverted T waves, especially in V_4 and other L chest leads, in a child more than 6 years who shows other evidence of RVH, indicates strain. Various drugs and metabolic changes can affect T waves and some of the more common of these are described later.

7. Ventricular Hypertrophy

(a) RVH

Difficult to diagnose in presence of RBBB. Also difficult to determine in child, less than 1 year of age. Criteria in child more than 1 year.

(i) Axis $> 120°$

(ii) R wave > 10mm in AVR, V_1

(iii) QR pattern in V_1

(b) LVH

(i) R wave in II, III > 45mm.

(ii) R wave in V_5, $V_6 > 30$mm.

(iii) S wave in V_1 or $V_2 > 25$mm.

Or sum of R + S in any of above leads if > 50mm.

8. Right Bundle Branch Block

Difficult to diagnose RVH in presence of RBBB
QRS prolonged > 0.1 sec.

The pattern in V_1 is similar to that seen in RVH – normally V_1 picks up only LV waves as the R wave is swamped. In RBBB conduction to RV is delayed so wave appears after LV wave.

In V_6 the RV may be seen as an S wave after the R.

R
T
V₆
Q   S

Causes include:
  Post surgery
  ASD secundum
  Ebsteins
  Myocarditis
  RV strain

9. Left Bundle Branch Block

Uncommon in children.
The majority are related to disorders of cardiac muscle –
e.g.   Cardiomyopathy
       Myocarditis
       Glycogenosis (Type IIA)

Changes best seen in V_1 and V_6.
In V_1 prolongation of the S wave can give a W-shaped wave
and in V_6 the R wave can be distorted to form an M. T wave
alterations are also observed.

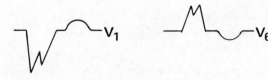

EFFECT OF DRUGS AND METABOLIC CHANGES ON ECG

1. Digitalis

Seen best II, III, aVF and R. chest leads.
Prolonged P-R interval
Shortening of QRS complex
S-T depression and T wave inversion
Virtually any arrhythmia
Bradycardia
Coupling – alternate normal beats with ectopics

2. Potassium

↑K$^+$ — absent P (initially seen as ↓ size and prolongation
    of P giving prolonged P-R interval)
    tall pointed T waves
    widening of QRS
↓K$^+$ — prolonged P-R interval
    flattening – absent T → T inversion
    depressed S-T segment
    tall U waves

3. Calcium

↓— prolongs rate corrected Q-T interval
↑— shortens rate corrected Q-T interval
    arrhythmias.

4. Tricyclic Antidepressants and Phenothiazines

See p.97 and 90.

RHEUMATIC FEVER

Aetiology
Post ß haemolytic strep. infection (only 50% give history of this).

Age Group
Very rare under 4 years. 5-15 years. Peak at 8. However much commoner and seen younger in some ethnic groups.

Diagnosis
Presence of 2 major criteria
or 1 major and 2 minor criteria

Note:
1. Except in patients with pure chorea, the absence of serological evidence of streptococcal infection in two or more antibody tests should stimulate a search for other possible diseases.
2. Elevated streptococcal antibody titres should never be basis of diagnosis of rheumatic fever, in absence of definitive clinical criteria.

Major Criteria
Carditis –   significant murmur
             cardiomegaly
             pericarditis
             congestive heart failure
             ECG changes (*see* p.17)
Polyarthritis
Chorea
Subcutaneous nodules
Erythema marginatum

Minor Criteria
Fever
Arthralgia (in absence of arthritis)

Prolongation of P-R interval (in absence of carditis)
Positive acute phase reactants – ESR, C-reactive protein;
leukocytosis
Past history of Rh fever or Rh heart disease

Supporting Evidence

Throat culture of group A ß haemolytic strep.

Other Findings of Significance

History of recent sore throat
Abdominal pain
Tachycardia
Epistaxis

Investigations

Throat swab and typing of streptococci
Blood screen and ESR
ASO titre, antistreptokinase titre, and antihyaluronidase titre
C-reactive protein
ECG
Chest X-ray

Notes:

1. ASOT positive in 70-85% only.
   Starts to rise approximately 1 week after sore throat.
   Maximum 3-5 weeks. Antistreptokinase and
   antihyaluronidase may be increased in absence of positive
   ASOT.
2. ECG
   Conduction — Prolongation of P-R interval not evidence
   of myocarditis – hence not related to
   prognosis
   Myocarditis — Prolongation of rate corrected Q-T interval.
   (Notched, flattened or inverted T waves not
   specific.)
   Pericarditis — Raised S-T segment.

Treatment

1. Penicillin (dose for age – *see* Pharmacopoeia).

Give for 10 days and thereafter indefinitely in prophylactic dose. (If allergic to penicillin, use erythromycin.)

2. Suppressive Agents

(a) If no carditis:
Aspirin (aim for blood level 25-35mg%).
Initially 100mg/kg/day, 6 divided doses, and then reduce by a third after three days and check blood levels.
Give for 7-14 days. Stop.
If persistence or recurrence – continue treatment till symptom-free for 7 days.

(b) If carditis (murmur, Q-T changes, Chest X-ray changes – cardiomegaly, pericarditis):
Prednisone may be used if actual or incipient myocardial failure is present. 2mg/kg/day – 4 divided doses. Give for 14 days, then taper off over next 4 weeks while reintroducing aspirin.

Note:

If CHF persists or reappears while decreasing prednisone, continue therapy with prednisone in full dosage for further 2-4 weeks. Then taper off while reintroducing aspirin as before.

The ESR is a simple and valuable guide to activity of rheumatic disease, and should be checked weekly.

3. Further Management

(a) Polyarthritis alone:

Hospital	No bedrest unless child elects
Home	After no symptoms for 72 hours
School	After no symptoms for 72 hours
Exertion	After 4 weeks without carditis developing
OPD	See weekly for first month ECG before each visit.

(b) Carditis without CHF:

Hospital	No bedrest but limited activity
Home	After carditis is stable (minimum stay of 2 weeks)
School	After 1 week at home

Exertion	After carditis is inactive for 1 month
OPD	See weekly until carditis is inactive for 6 weeks.

(c) Carditis with CHF:

Hospital	Bedrest until CHF is cleared
Home	After carditis is stable (minimum stay of 1 month)
School	After 2 weeks at home
Exertion	After carditis in inactive for 1 month
OPD	Follow at 1-week intervals until carditis is inactive for 2 months.

Prophylaxis

Penicillin V 250mg b.d. BEFORE MEALS for life.
If patient co-operation unreliable give benzathine penicillin 600 000-1 200 000 units (400-750mg) i.m. every 15-30 days.
Some would also consider tonsillectomy.
For dental treatment in those who have had carditis: add erythromycin 50mg/kg/day in 4 divided doses for 4 days starting 2 hours before the procedure.

THERAPY FOR PREVENTION OF SUBACUTE BACTERIAL ENDOCARDITIS

Endocarditis can occur in any form of mechanical heart disease, congenital or acquired.

When a congenital lesion is COMPLETELY repaired, the risk disappears. However, if even a trivial lesion remains then the risk is still there.

Prophylaxis

1. Good dental hygiene and $\frac{6}{12}$ dental appointments.
2. Antibiotic cover necessary for all dental procedures involving periodontal tissues and the gingivae, and for any procedure to the teeth where surrounding tissues are diseased. All tooth extractions must be covered.

   Antibiotic cover also for:
   Tonsillectomy and adenoidectomy

Bronchoscopy
Intubation of GI tract
Instrumentation of GU tract
Surgery of potentially infected areas
Potentially infected trauma
Obstetric deliveries
Focal sepsis

Dosage Schedule

Major Procedures

Benzylpenicillin 1 million units i.m.
— 1 hour before extraction
— evening of procedure
— next morning

Thereafter, penicillin V for 2-4 days in dose for age

Minor Procedures

< 5 years	Penicillin V 125mg 6-hourly for 4 days, starting 2 hours before procedure
5-12 years	Benzylpenicillin 250 000-500 000 units i.m. 1 hour before the procedure and 250mg penicillin V 6-hourly for 4 days, starting 4 hours after the procedure.
12 years +	Benzylpenicillin 1 megaunit i.m. 1 hour before the procedure and 500mg penicillin V orally, 6-hourly for 4 days, starting 4 hours after the procedure.

If the patient is unlikely to take oral medication reliably then
i.m. therapy: Mixture of benzylpenicillin and procaine
penicillin ($\frac{1}{2}$-1 megaunit of each) should be given once a day
for 3 doses, starting 1 hour before the procedure.

Major and Minor Procedures

When patients are taking continuous penicillin prophylaxis for
rheumatic fever, then erythromycin in a dose of 50mg/kg/day
should be given in 4 divided doses for 4 days starting 2 hours
before the procedure.

Child Abuse

There are various forms of child abuse – non-accidental injury; failure-to-thrive; neglect; sexual abuse; emotional deprivation. The type most likely to present acutely is non-accidental injury.

Non-Accidental Injury (NAI)

Inflicted injuries can be fractures, bruises, abrasions, incisions, burns, poisonings. Lacerations are rarely associated with NAI. Concomitant signs of neglect are present in a *minority* of cases.

Diagnosis

The diagnosis should be seriously considered in any of the following situations.

1. Any child under 2 years of age with a fracture.
2. Any child with multiple bruises.
3. Any unexplained injury.
4. Any injury which is unlikely to have occurred in the manner stated.
5. When the parent or caretaker offers different explanations to account for the injury.
6. Past history of frequent 'accidents' (note though that families whose children have frequent accidents often share similar characteristics with families whose children are abused).
7. Marked delay between injury and presentation for medical help.
8. Unusual or bizarre clinical presentations.
9. Repeated consultations for apparently trivial reasons.

There are certain findings which can be viewed as diagnostic of NAI. These would include pattern bruises, multiple fractures of different ages and some specific types of fracture.

Management

When NAI is suspected:
1. Notify the consultant on call.

2. Document history in minute detail so repeated interrogation is not needed to establish all the details of the parents' story as to how the injury occurred.
3. It is usually advisable to admit the child to hospital to ensure his or her immediate safety.
4. Physical examination should include inspection of inside of mouth (torn frenulum), optic fundi (retinal haemorrhages) and perineum for evidence of sexual abuse. Document all injuries precisely, recording for each, size, shape, colour and location.
5. Immediate investigations:
   platelet count and coagulation studies (if marked bruising);
   photographs (inform photographer they may be needed for legal purposes)
      black and white prints
      colour slides/prints;
   skeletal survey if child under 4 years of age. In older children X-ray only if clinical indication.
6. Medium and long term management can and should only be decided after the accumulation of data from a variety of sources. Details are outside the scope of this handbook.

Note:

Failure to make the diagnosis is usually because of inadequate levels of suspicion, although it may be impossible to establish the diagnosis on clinical findings alone. High rate of re-injury in unaltered situations. Prevention of physical re-injury is not of itself a good indication of success.

Chromosomes

The main usefulness of detecting a chromosomal abnormality lies in being able to:

1. Confirm a suspected clinical diagnosis, e.g. Down's.
2. Further investigate certain clinical problems (*see* below), and guide management.
3. Facilitate accurate genetic counselling.

A chromosomal analysis should be requested in these clinical situations:

1. Suspected Down's, trisomy 13, trisomy 18, Turner's.
2. Any dysmorphic infant ± congenital malformation(s) ± neurological problem.
3. Structural abnormality of internal or external genitalia and/or hypogonadism.
4. Malformed stillborn infant (intracardiac blood, or from IVC at autopsy; also discuss skin fibroblast culture with cytogenetics lab).
5. Worth considering in the screening of a child with developmental delay/mental retardation ± growth retardation.

Most labs are flexible in the amount of blood required when dealing with an infant. 1ml of heel-prick blood collected without clotting into a heparinised vessel should suffice (e.g. five $200\mu l$ capillary tubes). Allow 3-4 days for a preliminary result in urgent cases. In an emergency, a preliminary analysis may be done within a few hours on a bone marrow sample; discuss with lab.

Convulsions

EMERGENCY TREATMENT OF A CONVULSION

Drug Therapy

1. *Diazepam (Valium)*

   Initially: 0.25mg/kg/i.v. given over a 2-minute period.
   (Max 10mg)

Note:

When using diazepam observe closely patient's rate and depth of respiration as respiratory depression may be caused. *This is especially important if other anticonvulsants have already been given to the patient.*

Diazepam may conceal signs of meningeal irritation.

If child continues to convulse, or if seizures recur, and the patient has tolerated the injection without any respiratory embarrassment, give diazepam 0.4mg/kg/i.v. over 2 minutes. (Max. 15mg)

In the absence of adverse reactions a further dose of diazepam 0.5mg/kg i.v. over 2 minutes (max 20mg) may be given approximately 20 minutes after the second injection.

In practice it may be very difficult to give diazepam i.v. to some young children who are convulsing. In such situations consider rectal administration. Use undiluted diazepam i.v. solution (10mg/2ml). Administer via a short (6cm) length plastic tube with a blunt tip (e.g. portion of a feeding tube) and a 2ml plastic syringe. Inject fairly rapidly.

Dose:< 3 yrs 5-7mg (or 0.5-0.9mg/kg/dose)
     > 3 yrs 7.5-10mg (or 0.6-0.8mg/kg/dose)

Therapeutic blood levels are achieved within 4 mins. ± 1 min. If the convulsion has not ceased in 5 mins, this treatment may be repeated or i.v. diazepam given.

2. *Paraldehyde*

   0.15mg/kg/i.m.

Note:

This may be used after initial dose of diazepam and should be used if i.v. diazepam has produced respiratory depression.

3. If cerebral oedema is suspected:
   dexamethasone, 1.25mg/kg/stat i.v. or i.m. and then
   0.5mg/kg/day in four divided doses;
   mannitol, 2g/kg/i.v. over 30 mins.
4. Other anticonvulsants may also be used initially but only after discussion with the consultant.
   (a) Phenobarbitone.
       If weight less than 25kg – 6mg/kg/i.m. stat.
       If weight more than 25kg – 150mg/m^2/i.m. stat.
       Can be repeated after 1 hour and again after a further 4 hours if necessary.
   (b) Sodium amytal
       If weight less than 25kg – 5mg/kg/i.v.
       If weight more than 25kg – 125mg/m^2/i.v.
       Use 1% solution and give slowly over 4-5 mins.
       This dosage may be repeated up to a total of 4 times in the first 24 hours.
   (c) Phenytoin
       5-10mg/kg in saline i.v. over 15-30 mins. (Do not mix with dextrose solutions.)

Subsequent Therapy

If the initial convulsion has been severe and prolonged or if convulsions are repetitive, then after initial control has been achieved commence the following regimen:

Phenobarbitone i.m.
    Day 1 If weight less than 25kg – 6mg/kg/8-hourly
           If weight more than 25kg – 150mg/m^2/8-hourly
    Day 2 $\frac{2}{3}$ initial dose 8-hourly
    Day 3 $\frac{1}{3}$ initial dose 8-hourly

Note:

Again beware of respiratory depression if initial dose of phenobarbitone is given after i.v. diazepam.

EPILEPSY

BEWARE USING LABEL OF EPILEPSY IN CHILD WITH CONVULSIONS UNTIL POSITIVE OF DIAGNOSIS

General Principles of Drug Therapy

1. Avoid polytherapy. Use 1 drug at a time. Start with small doses and increase until control or therapeutic blood level is attained. Serum levels of all the more commonly used anticonvulsants are now available.
2. Only add another drug when maximum dose of previous drug has been reached, and only alter dose of one drug at any one time.
3. *Duration of therapy:* 3 years after last fit, but do not stop during puberty.
   e.g. *Method*:
   Decrease phenytoin over 1 month
   Then decrease phenobarbitone over next 2-3 months
   i.e. withdraw therapy slowly.

A.   Grand Mal (Tonic Clonic)

Investigations:

EEG

A/P and lateral skull X-ray

usually not necessary to perform these after first Grand Mal unless excessively prolonged (i.e. more than 10 minutes).

Brain scan should be considered – especially if there was a focal element to the convulsion, or if the EEG shows a definite asymmetry.

Drugs

1. Phenobarbitone – 3-10mg/kg/day in 2-3 divided doses.
   If (a) convulsions uncontrolled *or* (b) parents *volunteer* behaviour changes in child.
   then
2. Phenytoin (Dilantin) – 3-8mg/kg/day in 2-4 divided doses and decrease phenobarbitone in case of (b).
   If still uncontrolled, can increase doses separately until therapeutic levels achieved.

Side Effects:
  Phenobarbitone –
    Drowsiness, ataxia, irritability
  Phenytoin –
    Nystagmus
    Ataxia
    Drowsiness
    Gum hyperplasia
    Measles-like rash, lymphadenopathy, fever in 5%
    Hirsuitism in girls
    Obstinate constipation
    Decreased thyroid binding globulin
    therefore:
      decreased PBI
      decreased T_4
      increased T_3 resin uptake
    Megaloblastic anaemia
    Rickets

Note:

Phenobarbitone and certain other drugs can alter serum phenytoin level.

If Still Uncontrolled

3. Sodium valproate (Epilim) – 0-3 years 20-30mg/kg/day in 3 divided doses; 3-15 years 400mg/day in 3 divided doses and increase as necessary.

    Side Effects:
      Nausea
      Drowsiness
      Anorexia
      Hyperactivity
      Occasional hair loss
      Ataxia
      Marrow depression

4. Clonazepam (Rivotril) – 0.1-0.2mg/kg/day in 2 divided doses.

    Side Effects:
      Drowsiness
      Incoordination
      Bronchial hypersecretion
      Behaviour disturbances

5. Carbamazepine (Tegretol) – 10-30mg/kg/day in 2-4 divided doses.
   Introduce slowly to decrease incidence of side effects.

   > Side Effects:
   >> Drowsiness
   >> Nausea
   >> Unsteadiness
   >> Rarely marrow depression

6. Primidone (Mysoline) – 10-30mg/kg/day in 2-4 divided doses.

Note:

(a) Can make EEG worse; (b) early on can cause patient to present with acute abdomen; (c) give initially at bedtime.

   > Side Effects:
   >> Drowsiness
   >> Measles-like rash
   >> Ataxia which disappears rapidly
   >> Personality changes

7. Sulthiame (Ospolot) – 10-15mg/kg/day in 3 divided doses. Introduce gradually.

   > Side Effects:
   >> Initial tingling of extremities and face
   >> Tachypnoea
   >> Speech disturbances
   >> Reduced metabolism of phenytoin
   >> Toxic signs
   >> Hyperventilation

B. **Petit Mal (Absences)**

1. Classical – spike and wave at 3Hz (c.p.s.) on EEG

   Drugs:

   (a) Ethosuximide (Zarontin) – 15-50mg/kg/day in 2 divided doses.
       Introduce slowly to decrease incidence of side effects. May cause transient rash and photophobia which will disappear on temporary dose reduction.

       > Side Effects:
       >> Nausea/vomiting

Headache
Ataxia
Depression
Leukopenia and agranulocytosis – periodic
blood checks indicated
(b) Clonazepam (Rivotril) – 0.1-0.2mg/kg/day in
2 divided doses

Side Effects:
Drowsiness
Incoordination
Bronchial hypersecretion
Behaviour disturbances

(c) Sodium valproate (Epilim) – 0-3 years 20-
30mg/kg/day in 3 divided doses.
3-15 years 400mg/day in 3 divided doses and
increase as necessary.

Side Effects:
Nausea
Drowsiness
Anorexia
Hyperactivity
Occasional hair loss
Ataxia
Marrow depression

(d) Acetazolamide (Diamox) – 10-30mg/kg/day in
3 divided doses.

Side Effects:
Anorexia
Polyuria
Drowsiness
Paraesthesia
Rarely sulphonamide-type reactions –
fever
rash
Crystalluria
Renal calculus
Blood dyscrasia

2. *A typical Petit Mal*

Difficult to treat
Distinguished by:
(a) EEG spike and wave $1\frac{1}{2}$ or 5-6Hz (c.p.s.)

(b) Patient has recall of convulsion
Treatment as for Grand Mal. Try clonazepam (Rivotril) first.

C. Minor Motor Epilepsy

Difficult to control

Drugs

1. Nitrazepam (Mogadon) – 2.5mg nocte initially; increase to 0.15-2mg/kg/day in 2-3 divided doses, (wide range of tolerance).

    Side Effects:
    Drowsiness
    Ataxia
    Cough (due to increased bronchial secretions)
May be necessary to try a number of drugs:

2. Clonazepam (Rivotril) – *see* Grand Mal
3. Sodium valproate (Epilim) – *see* Grand Mal
4. Primidone (Mysoline) – *see* Grand Mal
5. Diazepam (Valium) – 2mg b.d. increasing up to 30mg/day
6. Phenytoin (Dilantin) – *see* Grand Mal
7. Ethosuximide (Zarontin) – *see* Petit Mal

FEBRILE CONVULSIONS

If there is any question in your mind of the possibility of
meningitis, then a lumbar puncture must be performed.
It is often difficult to separate simple benign febrile
convulsions from convulsions occuring with fever.
Generally speaking though the following points can be made
regarding simple benign febrile convulsions.

(a) No suggestion of focal element
(b) Duration less than 15 mins.
(c) No more than 2 seizures per febrile episode
(d) No more than 6 seizures within a year
(e) EEG normal 2-3 weeks after convulsion

Investigation

1. History
    FH of febrile convulsion
    PH of febrile convulsion
    system involved causing fever
2. Examination – source of fever
    ears
    throat
    chest
    urine
    exclude meningitis (by LP if indicated)
    blood pressure
3. Laboratory tests
    Nose and throat swabs for virology and bacteriology
    Urine for protein, microscopy and culture
    Chest X-ray
    Blood screen
    Other lab. tests may be indicated after discussion with
    consultant

Therapy

If convulsion prolonged for more than 10 minutes, treat as for
'convulsions' (p.24).

Otherwise:

1. Do not attempt vigorous reduction of temperature unless

more than 40°C.
2. If infection bacterial – e.g. signs on chest X-ray; increased w.b.c. with shift to left; otitis media – treat with penicillin or amoxycillin.
3. If child is having frequent febrile convulsions:
   EEG
   Consider prophylaxis with *rectal* diazepam:

Either

Give undiluted diazepam i.v. solution (10mg/2ml) rectally when rectal temperature is 38.5°C or above via a short (6cm) plastic tube with a blunt tip (e.g. a length of feeding tube) and a 2ml syringe. Inject fairly rapidly.
Dose: < 3 yrs: 5-7.5mg (or 0.5-0.9mg/kg/dose)
         > 3 yrs: 7.5-10mg (or 0.6-0.8mg/kg/dose)
Dose may be repeated every eight hours while temperature remains 38.5°C or above.

or

Diazepam suppository (5mg).
Give 5mg every eight hours while rectal temperature is 38.5°C or above.
Rectal injection of i.v. solution has more rapid action – therapeutic blood levels are achieved in 4 mins ± 1 min. May consider using this when child first develops fever and thereafter maintain on rectal suppositories for duration of febrile illness.
Continuous long-term prophylaxis with oral phenobarbitone is an alternative to rectal diazepam.
Parents may complain of behaviour change in child on phenobarbitone. May require drug to be stopped.

It is not necessary to treat the majority of benign febrile convulsions in the acute state with anticonvulsants. The majority will stop spontaneously within 10 minutes and will not recur.

Dermatology

Eczema

1. Avoid skin irritants
2. To prevent scratching
   — keep nails short
   — phenergan orally (*see* Pharmacopoeia)
3. Avoid using soap. Instead use emulsifying ointment as soap substitute.
4. Local therapy:
   (a) Remove crusts by bathing in emulsifying ointment and water. (Dissolve ointment in boiling water before adding to bath)
   If lesions are severely encrusted they will detach after soaking in warm light liquid paraffin.
   (b) Moist lesions – dry by repeated application of 20% sodium sulphate solution or copper and zinc sulphate lotion BPC
   (c) If not infected apply 1% hydrocortisone cream q.i.d. or more frequently initially if necessary.
   (d) When inflammatory reaction is settling apply oil of cade b.d. to limbs and cover with tube gauze.
   (e) To bring about final resolution apply tar preparation:
Liq. picis carb.	5%
Salicylic acid	3%
Hydrocortisone	1%
   Make up to 100% with soft yellow paraffin.
   (f) If appears infected:
   swab skin
   topical antibacterials t.d.s. (use neomycin or framycetin containing ointments)
   If severe – erythromycin orally. (*see* Pharmacopoeia)

Note:

Do not vaccinate child against smallpox.

Nappy Rash

1. Avoid irritants (e.g. fabric softeners)

2. Fully rinse detergents and soaps out of nappies.
3. Change nappy frquently. If possible have affected area exposed for periods.
4. Avoid plastic or rubber pants.
5. If persistent smell of ammonia on wet nappies soak dirty nappies in weak vinegar solution (1 cup/5l water).
6. Apply local protective medication
   e.g. Zinc and castor oil cream
      Karitane ointment:
Zinc oxide ung.	18.75%
Boric acid ung.	25%
Soya oil	25%
Yellow soft paraffin	to 100%
Beaten egg white	
7. 1% hydrocortisone cream may be used if inflammation is marked.

Secondary infection with *Candida albicans* may occur and is seen as whitish sodden scaling at the margin of the rash. Treat with gentian violet 0.5% or one of the proprietary creams/ointments.

Secondary bacterial infection is treated with neomycin or framycetin containing ointments after swabbing skin. If severe – oral erythromycin also.

Seborrhoeic Dermatitis

Apply dilute salicylic and sulphur ointment twice daily for a max. of 2 weeks for the mild rash.

Composition of ointment:
Salicylic acid	1%
Precipitated sulphur	1%
Lanoline	25%

Make up to 100% with soft yellow paraffin.

(For severe cases 1% hydrocortisone may be added)

If the scalp is severely affected then wash hair daily using any one of the numerous proprietary shampoos. Rinse thoroughly and apply castor oil to scalp. Leave until prior to next hair wash and then scrape scales off using hard edge of cardboard or a fine-tooth comb. After washing and rinsing apply dilute salicylic and sulphur ointment.

Impetigo

1. Avoid where possible contact with other children.
2. Segregate child's clothing etc. from rest of family.
3. Take skin swabs.
4. Bathe off crusts as they form with cetrimide 0.1% lotion or after soaking in warm light liquid paraffin.
   Moist lesions may be dried by repeated application of copper and zinc sulphate lotion BPC or 20% sodium sulphate solution.
   Extensive, ulcerated lesions respond to wet packs of Eusol (calcium hypochlorite solution) 1:4 dilution.
5. Apply topical antibiotics 4-6 times/day. Use neomycin or framycetin containing ointments (unless and until culture reports show resistant organisms present)
6. Oral erythromycin (*see* Pharmacopoeia) for 7 days.

Scabies

1. Hot bath, during which scrubbing, particularly between fingers, about wrists, navel and other affected areas is carried out.
2. Paint all skin surfaces from neck to toes with benzyl benzoate. This may produce some stinging so for young children use gamma benzene hexachloride 1% (Lorexane). After drying, repaint to ensure no area has been missed.
3. Change all clothing. Wash all removed articles, bedding etc. and hang in sun to dry.
4. 48 hours later repaint body again.
5. The patient should not bathe, wash or shower during the treatment.
6. 24 hours after the second painting another hot bath is taken. The course of treatment is then completed.

Head Lice

1. Wash hair thoroughly with soap and water. Dry.
2. Rub 1% gamma benzene hexochloride (Lorexane) cream well into affected skin and hair and also adjacent areas.
3. Do not wash the hair for 7-10 days.

One application should kill all the lice and prevent reinfestation for about three weeks.

Scalp Ringworm

1. Usually contracted from a cat or dog.
2. Griseofulvin 10-15mg/kg/day in two to four divided doses. Given in milk – 4-6 weeks' course
3. Apply benzoic acid ointment (Whitfield's) twice daily to affected area.

Note:

Treat ringworm of the body with half strength Whitfield's ointment applied twice daily to affected areas.

Diabetes Mellitus

MANAGEMENT OF PATIENT WITH
UNCONTROLLED DIABETES MELLITUS

1. Establish Diagnosis

History + hyperglycaemia ± ketoacidosis. (Remember glycosuria is not always due to diabetes mellitus).
If known diabetic, exclude hypoglycaemia (Dextrostix). If unsure give 1ml/kg of 50% dextrose i.v.

2. Initial Investigations

(a) Blood sugar and ketones (if sugar very high and no ketones consider hyperosmolar state).
(b) Electrolytes and urea, pH and bicarbonate.
(c) ? any precipitating factors – especially infection – blood screen; chest X-ray; urine culture

Remember ↑ WBC can occur in diabetic ketoacidosis even in absence of infection.

3. Establish Severity of Condition

i.v. therapy (stage 1, below) is essential if any of the following are present:
  Vomiting
  5% or greater dehydration (*see* p.48)
  Blood sugar > 17mmol/l
  Ketoacidosis
  Coma
Otherwise, rehydrate orally, using Stage 2 treatment regimen.

4. Initial Therapy
Stage 1
(a) Insulin

Either
Soluble insulin 0.1 unit/kg i.v. slowly as a bolus.
Then soluble insulin 0.1 unit/kg/hr i.v. until blood sugar <
12mmol/l.

The insulin is added to the drip chamber each hour and run
in over approx. 15 minutes.
Once the blood sugar < 12mmol/l change to the Stage 2
insulin regimen.

Blood sugar must be estimated hourly while using this regimen

Or (if the above regimen is not practicable)
Soluble insulin 0.1-0.5 unit/kg/i.m. stat. and then
subsequent doses at 4-6 hourly intervals depending on the
response which should be guaged by:
 (i) Dextrostix, or blood sugar if readily available.
(ii) Urine testing – if child is old enough to comply have
     him empty his bladder half an hour before urine test
     due, then test subsequent sample.

Subsequent doses of insulin calculated by using sliding
scale below – *This is a rough guide only*

	Dose in Units		
Urine Test	**< 4 years**	**4-10 years**	**Adolescent**
2%	d	d	d
1%	d – 1	d – 2	d – 3
¾%	d – 2	d – 3	d – 4
less than ¾%	nil	nil	nil
Acetone	Extra insulin (1-3 units) should be given for		
+ + or + + +	this amount of acetone provided there is ¾% or		
	more of glucose also present		
	d = initial dose of insulin given (0.1-0.5 unit/kg)		

(b) Rehydration:
   (i) 0.9% NaCl. In first hour at rate of 20ml/kg.
  (ii) Thereafter choice and rate of i.v. fluid based on aim
       to correct electrolyte imbalance and fluid deficit
       and provide maintenance over 24 hour period. (*see*
       p.48)
 (iii) 4% dextrose must be added to i.v. fluids once blood
       sugar falls below 13mmol/l.
 (iv) Supplements:
       —20mmol/l of KCl as soon as insulin given and
         urine output established.

—In severe cases when pH < 7.1 give HCO_3^- .
(*see* p.1)

Note:

In hyperosmolar coma:
1. Slower rate of rehydration (over 48 hours)
2. Delete 4% dextrose until blood sugar is normal
3. Do not give HCO_3^-

(c) Supportive therapy
  (i) In comatose patients use continuous gentle gastric suction. This may also be useful if patient continues to vomit.
  (ii) If clear evidence of bacterial infection treat vigorously with antibiotics.

Stage 2

Blood sugar falling (under 12mmol/l); ketosis diminishing; patient fully conscious and able to eat and drink.
(a) Re-establish oral feeding. Give small, frequent (approx. 4 hourly), relatively high carbohydrate meals and drinks.
(b) Maintain i.v. (using 0.18% NaCl + 4% dextrose) until feeding definitely re-established orally, but reduce infusion rate.
(c) Give soluble insulin s.c. 4 hourly based on urine testing. Calculate dose using sliding scale (p.38)

Stage 3

Patient stabilisation

1. *Aims*

(a) Normal growth and adolescence both physically and emotionally
(b) Avoid stringent rules for management and aim for family participation
(c) No restriction of activity
(d) Education of patient and family
(e) Avoid persistently high or wildly fluctuating blood glucose levels, ketoacidosis and hyperlipidaemia
(f) Avoid frequent or severe hypoglycaemia
(g) Avoid urinary frequency and/or nocturia

2. *Diet*

Enlist services of qualified dietician.

Approx. total energy requirement: 4.2 + 0.42MJ for each year of life (4.2MJ = 1000 kcal).

1g FAT	39.1kJ
1g CHO	17.6kJ
1g PROTEIN	16.8kJ

Optimal protein intake in child –

less than 3 years	3g/kg
more than 3 years	2g/kg

Avoid extra sugar

3. *Insulin*

Available insulin preparations:

Insulin Product	Strength (U/ml)	Action in Hours			Frequency of Administration	Origin
		Onset (hours)	Peak	Duration		
Insulin B.P.	20,40, 80,160, 300	$\frac{1}{2}$	2-4	6-8	Two or three times daily	Beef
Neutral mono-component insulin (Actrapid MC)	40,80	$\frac{1}{2}$	2-4	6-8	Two or three times daily	Pork
Insulin zinc suspension B.P. (Novo Semilente MC)	40,80	1	5-8	10-15	Twice daily	Pork
Mono-component biphasic insulin (Rapitard MC)	40,80	2	4-13	15-22	Twice daily (occasionally single dose adequate)	Pork and Beef
Neutral porcine mono-component insulin (Monotard MC)	40,80	2	7-14	15-22	Usually once daily (occasionally twice daily is necessary)	Pork

Insulin zinc suspension 'Lente' B.P. (Novo Lente MC)	40,80	2	7-14	18-24	Usually once daily (occasionally twice daily is necessary)	Pork and Beef
Insulin Isophane (NPH)	40,80, 160	2	8-10	28-30	Once daily	Pork or Beef
Protamme zinc Insulin B.P.	40,80	4-8	14-20	24-36	Once daily	Beef
Insulin zinc Suspension B.P. 'Ultra-Lente' (Novo Ultralente MC)	40,80	4-8	11-27	26-36	Once daily	Beef

U 100 Insulin (100 units per ml) is available in Australia, Canada and the United States. In New Zealand (as from 1 March 1981) all insulins other than protamine zinc insulin are available as U 100 Insulin.

After stabilisation on soluble insulin an attempt should be made to transfer the child to a regimen using longer acting insulins either in a single daily injection (given approximately 30 mins before breakfast) or on a b.d. basis. Initial total daily dose of longer acting insulin should be estimated as approximately $\frac{2}{3}$ of the daily dose of soluble insulin which was required to stabilise the child.
Generally best control achieved with insulin injection before breakfast and before evening meal, but dose, type(s) and timing must be individualised.
Modify dosage according to urine testing.

4. *Urine Tests*

Where possible, always have patient empty bladder half an hour before test due and then test second specimen.

For stabilisation –
   pre-breakfast
   pre-lunch
   pre-evening meal
   pre-bedtime

Then usually can achieve good control by monitoring pre-breakfast and pre-evening meal urines.
   After initial control not necessary routinely to test for

acetone – not always reliable in children.

Check for its presence if urines consistently more than 2% for more than 48 hours, or if child unwell.

Note:

If urines show persistent glycosuria yet patient has symptoms of hypoglycaemia –
or
if control seems to require constantly increasing doses of insulin –
then consider Somogyi phenomenon – in which case decrease insulin dose. Rising insulin requirements can occasionally be sign of resistance – defined as requirement greater than 2 units/kg/day.
A 24 hour collection of urine (or even better, 2 consecutive 12 hour collections) for the estimation of glucose output can be used as an aid to estimating the degree of control being achieved. Output should be less than 7% of daily intake of carbohydrate.

5. *Before Discharge*
   (a) Height and weight of child
   (b) Blood sugar series and urine tests for:
       (i) degree of control
       (ii) reliability of urine tests for that particular patient.
       Final control not achieved until patient is at home living normally.
   (c) Ensure parents have continuing contact with dietician
   (d) Ensure parents capable of drawing insulin up properly and giving the injection
   (e) Ensure parents are aware of different sites available for injection
   (f) Ensure parents can manage hypoglycaemic shock
   (g) Emphasise need to vary injection sites
   (h) Inform parents of:
       (i) signs and symptoms of hypoglycaemic shock
       (ii) situations that may lead to hyperglycaemia e.g. infection
       (iii) possibility that child's requirements may fall off over next 2-3 months before rising again
       (iv) Medic Alert service

Ear, Nose & Throat

EAR PROBLEMS

Do not syringe or attempt to remove a foreign body or wax unless you are sure of yourself. Ask for expert help rather than risk hurting the child.
There is rarely any hurry to remove a foreign body.

Otitis Externa

May be secondary to otitis media

Treatment
1. Clean meatus of discharge as required, by dry mopping or suction. Send specimen to bacteriology.
2. Antibiotic/steroid drops q.i.d. after mopping (e.g. betamethasone – neomycin preparation). If inpatient, a wick of ½ inch ribbon gauze impregnated with the solution can be used. Change b.d.
3. Keep ear dry
4. Check for underlying otitis media
5. Continue therapy until condition completely resolved

Acute Otitis Media

Remember a crying child may have a moderately injected drum.

Treatment
1. If child vomiting or not feeding give parenteral antibiotics.
2. Amoxycillin is drug of first choice. Give dose for age (*see* Pharmacopoeia) for 7 days.
3. If no response to amoxycillin after 24 hours then assume infection due to resistant haemophilus or staphylococcus, and treat with cloxacillin. (*see* Pharmacopoeia)
4. If ear has perforated, clean discharge frequently.
5. *NB* Ear should be examined after completion of antibiotic course.

Complications

1. Glue ear
   May follow acute otitis media or arise apparently *de novo*.
   Very common. Presents as deafness or with educational
   problems. Occasionally some otalgia. Drum may appear
   normal to superficial inspection. Refer if symptoms persist –
   surgical problem.
2. Chronic perforation
   (a) Clear out discharge if present
   (b) Glycerine: Ichthyol drops q.i.d. or on wick if inpatient.
       (Most topical antibiotics are ototoxic)
   (c) Refer to ENT surgeon for consideration of repair.

Frequently Recurrent Otitis Media

1. Consider prolonged (6-12 weeks) amoxycillin therapy.
2. If this is unsuccessful, problem can be relieved by insertion
   of ventilation tubes – can be done even in first year of life if
   problem very severe.
3. Role of adenoids disputed. There is little scientific evidence
   to support adenoidectomy for recurrent otitis media, and
   adenoids are rarely significantly enlarged in first two years
   of life. Nonetheless most ENT surgeons remove adenoids if
   large.

NASAL PROBLEMS

Foreign Body

Refer to experienced person unless convinced you can remove
easily first time without hurting child.

Epistaxis

Treatment

1. Sit patient up
2. Compress nose as shown until bleeding stops
3. Do not pack without expert instruction
4. Severe prolonged epistaxis should be managed by expert,
   not by amateur pack

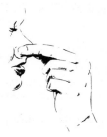

5. Vast majority due to rupture of small vessel on ant. nasal septum, but may occasionally be associated with a general bleeding disorder, childhood exanthems, or rheumatic fever.

Acute Purulent Rhinitis

Treatment

Penicillin in dose for age after taking swab
    If unilateral, offensive purulent discharge may indicate a foreign body.

Allergic Rhinitis

Treatment

1. If feasible, remove any precipitating factors
2. Antihistamines (*see* Pharmacopoeia). Drowsiness may make these drugs unacceptable and they are not always effective.
3. If not improved – sodium cromoglycate (Rynacrom) spray
4. If not improved – beclomethasone nasal spray. (Beware of long term use since long term effects not yet fully determined).

THROAT PROBLEMS

Acute Tonsillitis

General
1. May be bacterial (usually streptococcal) or viral.
2. Clinical examination does not necessarily differentiate between the two.
3. Laboratory results of value in retrospect.

Treatment
Penicillin in dose for age (*see* Pharmacopoeia)
If throat swab negative, stop treatment.
If haemolytic streptococci cultured, continue for 10 days.

Tonsillectomy

General
1. No uniform agreement as to indications for surgery.
2. Mere physical size of tonsils is of little importance.
3. In assessing situation a reliable history of recurrent sore throats which respond to penicillin is of more value than clinical examination.
4. The age of the child is of importance:
   (a) It is questionable if there is any justification for surgery before the age of 2.
   (b) In the under-3 years group, the indications must be overwhelming.
   (c) Very strong indications are needed to suggest surgery in the under-5 years age group.

The indications for surgery in the under-fives may be summarised as a failure of adequate conservative management in the presence of severe symptoms which continue over a period. Two or three sore throats a year which respond to antibiotics are not an indication; if more frequent symptoms occur, it is reasonable to:
(a) Look elsewhere in the family for a source of infection and
(b) Maintain the child on long-term penicillin as for rheumatic fever prophylaxis. This will often enable surgery to be postponed until the child is more able to withstand it.
   It is difficult to reach any sort of rational decision without observing the child over a period of months, if not years.

Sore throats often diminish in frequency and severity
during this period of observation.
(c) Children over 5 years.
Recurrent episodes of tonsillitis, persisting over years and
resulting in significant loss of time at school, is the
principal indication.

Post Tonsillectomy Bleed

Management
1. If within 24 hours treat seriously:
   (a) erect i.v.
   (b) Cross-match 1 unit of blood
   (c) Close observations
   (d) Notify surgeon
2. After 1 week:
   Usually trivial but admission to hospital advised (if only for
   parents' peace of mind)
   Give penicillin in dose for age (*see* Pharmacopoeia).

Fluid & Electrolyte Balance

Maintenance

Weight		ml/kg	K$^+$ mmol/kg
Newborn < 1.5kg	Day 1	90	1.5
	Day 2	120	1.5
	Day 3	160	1.5
> 1.5kg	Day 1	60	1
	Day 2	90	1
	Day 3	120	1
kg 4-10 ⎫		100 minus	⎧ 2.5
10-20 ⎬		(Age in	⎨ 2
20-40 ⎭		years × 3)	⎩ 1.5

Amount may need to be increased in hot weather or with fever.

Dehydration

1. Calculation of deficit:

    (a) Of H_2O
    5% dehydrated – 50ml/kg
    10% dehydrated – 100ml/kg   (% loss of body
    15% dehydrated – 150ml/kg   weight *see* p.51)

    (b) Of sodium   a = Serum Na$^+$ level

    Calculate Na deficit as follows:
    $(142-a) \times {}^{65}/_{100} \times$ wt. in kg.
    Therefore No. of ml of 0.9% NaCl necessary
    $= (142-a) \times {}^{65}/_{100} \times$ wt. in kg $\times {}^{1000}/_{154}$
    1 l of 0.9% NaCl contains 154mmol/Na$^+$

    (c) Of chloride   b = Serum Cl$^-$ level

    Calculate deficit as follows:
    $(103-b) \times {}^{65}/_{100} \times$ wt. in kg.
    No. of ml of 0.9% NaCl to correct deficit
    $= (103-b) \times {}^{65}/_{1000} \times$ wt. in kg $\times {}^{1000}/_{154}$
    1 l of 0.9% NaCl contains 154mmol/Cl$^-$

    (d) Of potassium
    Replace max. of 3mmol/kg/day

Notes:
1. Rate should not be greater than 0.5mmol/kg/hr
2. Deficiency requires correction for 4-5 days
3. Ensure satisfactory renal output before giving potassium solutions

2. For continuing excessive losses due to aspirate or diarrhoea refer to table below

Approximate electrolyte composition of gastrointestinal fluids mmol/l

Fluid	Na^+	K^+	Cl^-	H^+	HCO_3^-
Gastric	140	15	150	80	0
Small intestine	130	15	120	0	30
Pancreatic	135	15	100	0	50
Diarrhoeal	40	40	40	0	40

3. Rate of replacement

This will depend on what the electrolyte results reveal. Commence as for isotonic dehydration and modify as necessary

ISOTONIC dehydration. Deficit given over 48-hour period

Day 1 (D_1): Maintenance with
   0.18% NaCl and 4% dextrose
   + K^+ after renal output established
   + $\frac{1}{2}$ of calculated deficit (as 0.18% NaCl with 4% dextrose)
   + Excessive continuing losses e.g. severe diarrhoea

Note:
To maximum of 1 l if child less than 1 year old.

Day 2 (D_2): Maintenance
   + Remaining deficit
   + Excessive continuing losses

Thereafter: Maintenance + losses

HYPONATRAEMIC dehydration (Serum $Na^+ < 130$mmol)

As for Isotonic except give calculated amount of Na^+ deficit in D_1 as 0.9% saline

HYPERNATRAEMIC dehydration (Serum $Na^+ > 150$mmol)

Deficit should be corrected slowly
D_1: *Maintenance with*
   0.18% NaCl and 4% dextrose
   + K^+ after renal output established
   + $\frac{1}{3}$ deficit as 0.18% NaCl and 4% dextrose
   + losses

D_2 and D_3 as D_1
Thereafter: Maintenance + losses.

Gastroenteritis

Vomiting and diarrhoea are frequent presenting symptoms in a variety of conditions apart from primary gastroenteritis, e.g. otitis media, pneumonia, meningitis, urinary tract infection, appendicitis.

Underlying infection in other systems should be considered in cases of D & V but equally, symptoms in other systems do not exclude the presence of primary gastrointestinal infection.

Note:

Repeated vomiting with little or no diarrhoea is rarely due to gastroenteritis.

MANAGEMENT

1. Estimate Degree of Dehydration

by estimating % loss of body weight. Best guide is present weight compared with known weight before onset of illness.

5% fretful
    marked thirst
    feeds eagerly but often vomits
    loss of skin turgor

10% irritability more marked
    eyes sunken
    inappropriate tachycardia
    extremities cold
    may be overbreathing (metabolic acidosis)

15% peripheral circulatory failure
    body cold
    extremities cyanosed
    desire to suck lost
    fontanelle deeply sunken
    cornea may be glazed and eyes rolled up.

If more than 5% dehydration or if vomiting prominent then rehydrate i.v.

(*see* fluid and electrolyte therapy – p.48)

Notes:

(a) If previous weight unknown, standard growth charts may be used to check clinical assessment of weight loss.

(b) If 12% dehydrated commence with plasma or 0.9% saline (whichever is most readily available).
Give 20ml/kg in 1 hour.

(c) In exceptional circumstances
(if drip difficult to erect and child is severely shocked).
While ongoing attempts are being made to erect a drip infuse 20ml/kg of 0.9% saline stat, intraperitoneally, using a 23 guage needle attached to drip and introduced in midline approximately 2.5cm below umbilicus. As needle passes below skin, turn drip full on and advance needle until drip runs freely.

2. Investigations

(a) Faeces for bacterial culture and sensitivity and where possible virus identification by electron microscopy, enzyme-linked immunosorbent assay (ELISA) or culture.

(b) Electrolytes and urea

(c) Blood screen

Notes:

(a) Virus identification techniques are not available in many centres. Viruses such as rotavirus and the Norwalk agent are the most common cause of gastroenteritis in children, particularly in winter and early spring. It would be justifiable to send specimens to a virus laboratory for identification from the first few cases in an epidemic outbreak to establish the aetiology.

(b) Virus excretion is most profuse from the second to fourth day after onset of diarrhoea.

(c) It is very difficult to identify viruses as a cause of diarrhoea once the stool has become formed again.

Gastroenteritis is highly infectious. Strict isolation is essential until

(i) The child is back onto full diet without symptoms
or

(ii) Seven days from onset of the gastroenteritis – whichever is the shorter period.

3. Oral Therapy

(a) Initial – use ward gastroenteritis solution
Suggested composition:

dextrose	50g
sodium chloride	1.7g
potassium bicarb.	2.3g
water	1000ml

The mixture is usually stored as a dry powder, the 1000ml water being added just before use.

(b) After 24-48 hours or when frequency of stools decreases:
Half strength milk formula. In cases which relapse, consider disaccharide intolerance.

(c) After a further 24 hours – if no deterioration – full strength feeds for 24 hours and then discharge.

Note:

Milk intolerance due to secondary disaccharidase deficiency is a common complication of gastroenteritis in young infants (*see* below). Because of this it may be advisable to commence 'milk' feeds with non-lactose-containing formulae in young infants who have had gastroenteritis (*see* list on page 77). Rice (not made with milk), unsweetened apple sauce and banana are suitable initial solids for older children.
Early nutrition may help repair the damaged intestinal mucosa.

4. Complications

Secondary Sugar Intolerance: Lactose intolerance is common in small infants following gastroenteritis. It can be expected in up to 50% of those under 6 months but in less than 10% of those 6-12 months of age.

Diagnosis
Line the napkins with a thin sheet of plastic to collect the fluid portion of the stool. A small volume of fluid stool is diluted with twice its volume of water, and 15 drops of this suspension tested with a 'Clinitest' in an Ames' test-tube. A result of $\frac{1}{4}\%$ or less is regarded as negative, $\frac{1}{4}$-$\frac{1}{2}\%$ considered suspect, and more than $\frac{1}{2}\%$ indicates the presence of abnormal amounts of sugar or reducing substances.

Management

If $\frac{1}{2}\%$ or more is present on two occasions, a low lactose formula should be introduced (*see* list on page 00).

If there are significant amounts of reducing substances present in faeces while the infant is on a disaccharide-free formula, then secondary monosaccharide intolerance (a rare disorder) should be suspected. Manipulations of monosaccharide content, beyond the scope of this handbook, are required.

Secondary lactose intolerance may be present for a few days up to several months. Generally, the younger the infant, the longer the persistence of intolerance. A regime grading back to a milk formula should be tried after 1 week and then at monthly intervals.

Grading Over

Substitute 30ml of milk formula for 30ml of lactose-free formula in each bottle for 1-2 days. If no diarrhoea or vomiting occurs replace a further 30ml of lactose-free formula in each bottle with milk formula. Continue in this manner changing every 1-2 days until the daily intake is milk formula only.

If diarrhoea or vomiting occurs go back to total lactose-free formula feeding and try again in one month.

Note that it is dangerous suddenly to give a whole bottle of milk formula to an infant with possible lactose intolerance.

5. Kaolin, Opiates and Anti-Emetics

There is no evidence that kaolin mixtures help infants with gastroenteritis. Kaolin may increase the penetrance of some enteroviruses into the cell wall. Opiates and anti-emetics have *no place* in the treatment of gastroenteritis of infancy and early childhood. In particular DO NOT give diphenoxylate hydrochloride (Lomotil) to children as it can cause fatal respiratory depression.

6. Antibiotics

Antibiotics have no place in the treatment of virus gastroenteritis and diarrhoea due to enterotoxin producing strains of *E. coli* and *Salmonella*.

As a general rule, antibiotics should be given if there is evidence of the invasive nature of the organism e.g. a positive blood culture, or blood and pus cells in the stools (but consider the possibility of intussusception).

Growth and Development

GROWTH CURVES

Curves are compiled from data obtained in Australia and New Zealand. They are thus applicable to UK and other similarly constituted populations.

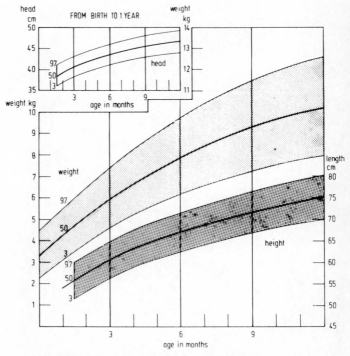

Weight, length and head circumference against age, during the first year of life (indicating 3rd, 50th and 97th percentiles).

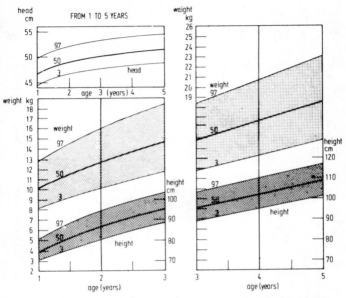

Weight, length and head circumference against age, first five years of life.

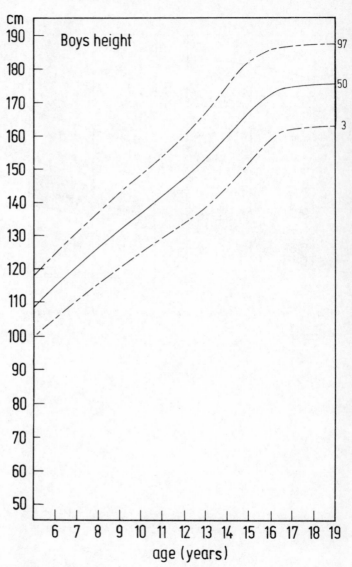

Height for age (boys)

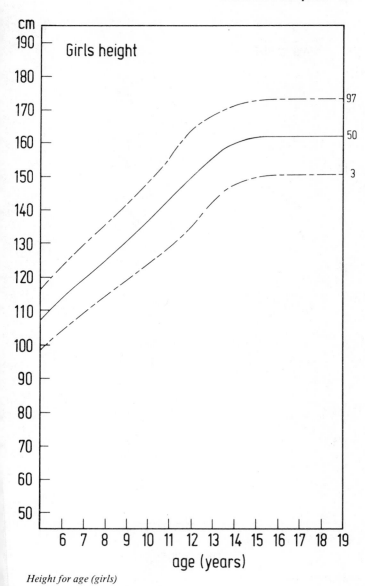

Height for age (girls)

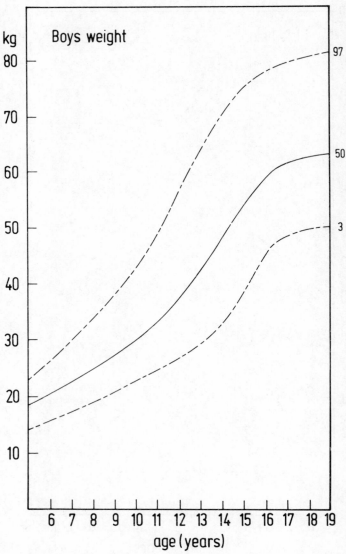

Weight for age (boys)

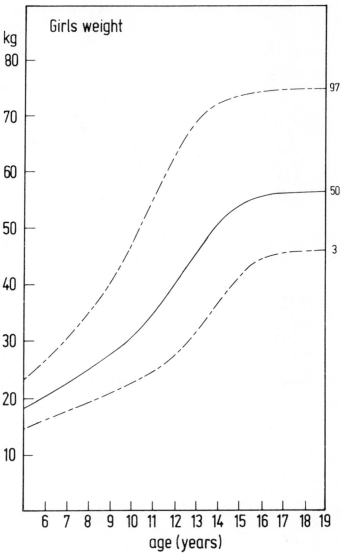

Weight for age (girls)

USUAL DEVELOPMENTAL MILESTONES

Month	1	Hears, sees
	$1\frac{1}{2}$	Smiles
	2	Lifts head in prone position
	3	Hand regard
	3-6	Lifts head in supine position
		Follows with eyes
		Reciprocation – helps in sitting up by lifting head in anticipation
	6	Loses hand regard
		Grasps and transfers
	7-9	Sits unsupported
		Crawls
		Lifts objects with finger and thumb
	10	Pulls himself up
		Imitates bye-bye
	11	Stands
	12	Walks with support
		Two appropriate words
	15-18	Walks well without support
		Feeds himself with cup

Note:

1. The above is only a rough guide. Many normal children are slow reaching SOME of these milestones.
2. A premature baby will usually be behind in achieving his milestones by the number of weeks he was premature.

SURFACE AREA

Height in centimetres

Height in inches

| 195 — 76 |
| 190 — 74 |
| — 72 |
| 180 — 70 |
| — 68 |
| 170 — 66 |
| — 64 |
| 160 — 63 |
| — 62 |
| — 61 |
| — 60 |
| 150 — 59 |
| — 58 |
| — 57 |
| — 56 |
| 140 — 55 |
| — 54 |
| — 53 |
| 130 — 52 |
| — 51 |
| — 50 |
| — 49 |
| — 48 |
| 120 — 47 |
| — 46 |
| 115 — 45 |
| — 44 |
| 110 — 43 |
| — 42 |
| — 41 |
| 105 — 40 |
| 100 — 39 |
| — 38 |
| 95 — 37 |
| — 36 |
| 90 — 35 |
| — 34 |
| 85 — 33 |
| — 32 |
| 80 — 31 |
| — 30 |
| 75 — 29 |
| — 28 |
| 70 — 27 |
| — 26 |
| 65 — 25 |
| — 24 |
| 60 — 23 |
| — 22 |
| 55 — 21 |
| — 20 |
| 50 — 19 |
| — 18 |
| 45 — 17 |
| — 16 |
| 40 |

Surface area in square meters

| 2 40 |
| 2 3 |
| 2 2 |
| 2 1 |
| 2 0 |
| 1 9 |
| 1 8 |
| 1 7 |
| 1 6 |
| 1 5 |
| 1 4 |
| 1 3 |
| 1 2 |
| 1 1 |
| 1 05 |
| 1 00 |
| 0 95 |
| 0 90 |
| 0 85 |
| 0 80 |
| 0 75 |
| 0 70 |
| 0 65 |
| 0 60 |
| 0 55 |
| 0 50 |
| 0 45 |
| 0 40 |
| 0 35 |
| 0 30 |
| 0 25 |
| 0 20 |
| 0 19 |
| 0 18 |
| 0 17 |

Weight in kilograms

Weight in pounds

| 110 — 250 |
| 100 |
| 90 — 200 |
| 80 |
| 70 — 150 |
| 60 |
| 50 |
| 45 — 100 |
| 40 — 90 |
| — 85 |
| 35 — 80 |
| — 75 |
| — 70 |
| 30 — 65 |
| — 60 |
| 25 — 55 |
| — 50 |
| 20 — 45 |
| — 40 |
| 15 — 35 |
| — 30 |
| — 25 |
| 10 0 |
| 9 0 — 20 |
| 8 0 |
| 7 0 — 15 |
| 6 0 |
| 5 0 |
| 4 5 — 10 |
| 4 0 — 9 |
| 3 5 — 8 |
| — 7 |
| 3 0 |

DENVER DEVELOPMENTAL SCREENING TEST (D.D.S.T.)

This is appropriate for children from birth to six years.

The 105 items are arranged in four sectors:
Personal – Social
Fine Motor – Adaptive
Language
Gross Motor.

Across the top and bottom of the test form are age scales which show ages in months from 1 to 24 and in years from $2\frac{1}{2}$ to 6. Each of the test items is represented on the form by a bar which is placed between the age scales to show when 25%, 50%, 75% and 90% of normal children can do that item.
Some test items have a small number on the left end of the bar, short instructions are given for these numbered items on p.66-7. Test items with an R on the bar are those which may be passed by report of the parent. Where possible the examiner should observe the child perform the item.
One hundred percent of normal children pass the item 'Equal Movements' at birth; this is indicated by a * at the end of the bar. The items 'Defines Words' and 'Composition of . . .' are passed by only 87% of normal children at 6.3 years.

General Instructions

1. Draw a line vertically across the chart at the point indicating the child's age.
2. Suggested order of testing follows the test form, but flexibility is permitted.
3. Begin each sector by giving the child tasks he can perform easily.
   Continue testing until the child fails three items in each sector. Usually there should be at least three passes to the left of any failure. All items passing through the age time should be attempted.
4. Allow the child three trials to perform each item if necessary before recording a failure. Some items require a specific number of trials; these are indicated on the test form. e.g. Catches Bounced Ball/2 of 3.

Item Scoring

Each item is scored on the bar near the 50% hatch mark. The items are scored:

P   *for* Pass
F   *for* Failure
R   *for* Refusal
NO *for* No opportunity for the child to perform the item.

Interpretation

A *delay* is any item failed which is completely to the left of the age line. That is, the child failed an item which 90% of children can pass at a younger age.

Delays on the test form are emphasised by colouring the right end of the bar of the delayed item.

Abnormal	2 or more sectors with 2 or more delays.
or	1 sector with 2 or more delays plus 1 or more sectors with 1 delay and in that same sector no passes intersecting the age line.
Questionable	1 sector with 2 or more delays.
or	1 or more sectors with 1 delay and in that same sector no passes intersecting the age line.
Untestable	When refusals occur in numbers large enough to cause the test result to be questionable or abnormal if they were scored as failures.
Normal	Any condition not listed above.

Instructions for numbered items on test form

1. Try to get child to smile by smiling, talking or waving to him. Do not touch him.
2. When child is playing with toy, pull it away from him. Pass if he resists.
3. Child does not have to be able to tie shoes or button in the back.
4. Move yarn slowly in an arc from one side to the other, about 6in above child's face. Pass if eyes follow 90° to midline. (Past midline; 180°)
5. Pass if child grasps rattle when it is touched to the backs or tips of fingers.
6. Pass if child continues to look where yarn disappeared or tries to see where it went. Yarn should be dropped quickly from sight from tester's hand without arm movement.
7. Pass if child picks up raisin with any part of thumb and a finger.

8. Pass if child picks up raisin with the ends of thumb and index finger using an over-hand approach.
9. Pass any enclosed form. Fail continuous round motions.

10. Which line is longer? (Not bigger.) Turn paper upside down and repeat. (3/3 or 5/6)

11. Pass any crossing lines.

12. Tell child to copy first. If failed, demon-strate.

When giving items 9, 11 and 12, do not name the forms. Do not demonstrate 9 and 11.

13. When scoring, each pair (2 arms, 2 legs, etc.) counts as one part.
14. Point to picture and tell child to name it. (No credit is given for sounds only.)

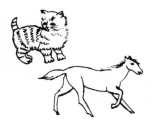
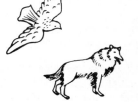

15. Tell child to: Give block to Mummy; put block on table; put block on floor. Pass 2 of 3.
    (Do not help child by pointing, moving head or eyes.)
16. Ask child: What do you do when you are cold? . . . hungry? . . . tired? Pass 2 of 3.
17. Tell child to: Put block *on* table; *under* table; *in front* of chair, *behind* chair.
    Pass 3 of 4. (Do not help child by pointing, moving head or eyes.)
18. Ask child: If fire is hot, ice is . . . ?; Mother is a woman, Dad is a . . . ?; a horse is big, a mouse is . . . ?. Pass 2 of 3.
19. Ask child: What is a ball? . . . lake? . . . desk? . . . house? . . . banana? . . . curtain? . . . ceiling? . . . hedge? . . . pavement? Pass if defined in terms of use, shape, what it is made of or general category (such as banana is fruit, not just yellow). Pass 6 of 9.
20. Ask child: What is a spoon made of? . . . a shoe made of? . . . a door made of? (No other objects may be substituted.) Pass 3 of 3.
21. When placed on stomach, child lifts chest off table with support of forearms and/or hands.
22. When child is on back, grasp his hands and pull him to sitting. Pass if head does not hang back.
23. Child may use wall or rail only, not person. May not crawl.
24. Child must throw ball overhand 3 feet to within arm's reach of tester.
25. Child must perform standing broad jump over width of test sheet. (8½ inches)
26. Tell child to walk forward,

    ∞∞∞∞→   heel within 1 inch of toe.
    Tester may demonstrate. Child must walk 4 consecutive steps, 2 out of 3 trials.
27. Bounce ball to child who should stand 3 feet away from tester. Child must catch ball with hands, not arms, 2 out of 3 trials.
28. Tell child to walk backward,

    ←∞∞∞∞   toe within 1 inch of heel.
    Tester may demonstrate. Child must walk 4 consecutive steps, 2 out of 3 trials.

Date and Behavioural Observations
(How child feels at time of test, relation to tester, attention span, verbal behaviour, self-confidence, etc.)

Haematology

Haematological values (venous unless otherwise stated)

Haemoglobin

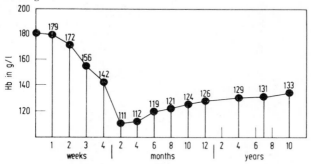

Venous and heel prick specimens cannot be directly compared. Errors are greater with *heel prick* specimens, and the value obtained is *higher* than for venous specimens.

Normal Cord Blood Values of Full Term Infants (Mean)

Hb 168g/l
Hct 0.53
r.b.c. 5.25×10^{12}/l
MCV 107fl
MCH 34pg
MCHC 317g/l
Reticulocytes 3%-7% ($100-300 \times 10^9$/l approx.)
Nucleated r.b.c's 0-24 (mean 7) per 100 leucocytes.
Platelets 290×10^9/l

Notes on neonates:

(a) The reticulocyte count falls to normal levels after the first week and later to subnormal levels until 4-8 weeks of age.

(b) The reticulocytes, and nucleated r.b.c's are increased with haemolysis, haemorrhage (fetal, or feto-maternal) and hypoxaemia.

(c) The platelet count may be reduced in premature infants in the first few weeks of life, occasionally $< 50 \times 10^9$/l but is not usually associated with bleeding problems.

Leukocyte values

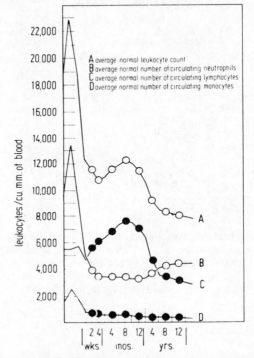

Age	Mean	95% range $\times 10^9$/l	
Birth	18.1	9.0-30.0	70% neutrophil series
2 weeks	11.4	5.0-20.0	40% neutrophil series
8 months	12.2	6.0-17.5	30% neutrophil series
1 year	11.4	6.0-17.5	30% neutrophil series
4 years	9.1	5.5-15.5	45% neutrophil series
10 years	8.1	4.5-13.5	60% neutrophil series

Notes:

(a) Some laboratories report the late unsegmented
    neutrophilic cells as (i) metamyelocytes or (ii) band or stab
    cells, depending on their degree of maturation. Other
    laboratories report them all as metamyelocytes.
(b) The *absolute* number of each cell type is of greater
    importance than the %.
(c) Atypical lymphocytes and Turk cells suggest an infective
    process, usually viral, or possibly a hypersensitivity
    process. Numerous atypical lymphocytes suggest infectious
    mononucleosis.
(d) Transient neutropenia may be seen in some viral infections.

Anaemias
Classification
    (i) Decreased effective r.b.c. production; deficiency states.
        e.g. Iron, B_{12}, folate, Vit. C deficiency
        Chronic disorders
        Marrow replacement
        Aplasia
      – Reticulocyte count *low*
        Some show blood film morphological changes.
    (ii) Haemorrhage
      – Reticulocytes *increased*, unless iron deficiency or
        other factors depressing erythropoiesis.
    (iii) Haemolysis
      – Reticulocytes *increased*.
        Some show r.b.c. morphological changes.
        Unconjugated bilirubin and urinary urobilinogen
        increased.
If an undiagnosed anaemic patient is to be transfused, obtain
adequate specimens for investigation *before* transfusion is given.
    (i) Full blood screen with blood film examination
    (ii) Reticulocyte count if no evidence of aetiology is
        present.
        If the reticulocytes are increased, perform direct
        Coombs' (antiglobulin) test and other investigations
        suggested from blood film and clinical history, e.g.
        osmotic fragility, autohaemolysis, r.b.c. enzyme
        studies, haemoglobin studies.
        If the reticulocytes are normal or decreased in an
        anaemic patient there is a hypoproliferative disorder.
        Check for primary or secondary causes.

Notes on neonates:

(a) *See* diagram opposite.
(b) Transfusion of infants (up to 6 months of age) – a blood specimen from the mother is required for crossmatching, in addition to a specimen from the infant.
(c) At delivery some fetal red cells usually enter the maternal circulation. The amount of feto-maternal blood exchange can be estimated by the Kleihauer test which counts the proportion of fetal to maternal cells in the maternal blood.
(d) Heparinised blood is often used for transfusion of infants to avoid hypocalcaemia induced by citrate. This blood can only be stored by a blood bank up to 24 hours.
(e) Haemostasis – neonates show:
Normal whole blood clotting times, platelet counts, Factor V, Factor VIII and fibrinogen.
The prothrombin time is usually *mildly* to moderately prolonged and the Vitamin K-dependent factors (II, VII, IX and X) are variably reduced. Factor XI may also be reduced.
The Vitamin K-dependent factors will revert to normal within 24-36 hours of giving Vitamin K, if liver function is normal.

Investigation of bleeding disorder:

(a) Clinical history
(b)   (i) Blood film, platelet count
     (ii) Fibrinogen (or thrombin clotting time), FDPs.
     These will indicate whether the defibrination syndrome is likely.
     (iii) Prothrombin time, PTTK, Factor assays if available

Blood volume

Neonate: 85ml/kg (mean)
After first month: 75ml/kg

Blood Transfusion

(a) Whole blood required in ml =
$$\frac{\text{Hb required } - \text{ Hb actual} \times \text{Wt in kg} \times 75\text{ml}}{\text{Hb required}}$$

Use 85 if < 1 month of age
(b) Packed cells: 2ml/kg will increase Hb by 10g/l

AN APPROACH TO THE DIFFERENTIAL DIAGNOSIS OF ANAEMIA IN THE NEWBORN

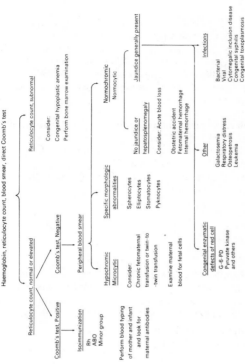

History - family, maternal and obstetric

Haemoglobin, reticulocyte count, blood smear, direct Coomb's test

Reticulocyte count, normal or elevated

Coomb's test, Positive

Isoimmunization
Rh
ABO
Minor group

Perform blood typing of mother and infant and look for maternal antibodies

Coomb's test, Negative

Peripheral blood smear

Hypochromic Microcytic

Consider:
Chronic fetomaternal transfusion or twin-to -twin transfusion

Examine maternal blood for fetal cells

Specific morphologic abnormalities

Spherocytes
Elliptocytes
Stomatocytes
Pyknocytes

Congenital enzymatic defects of red cell

G, 6, PD
Pyruvate kinase and others

Reticulocyte count, subnormal

Consider:
Congenital hypoplastic anemia
Perform bone marrow examination

Normochromic Normocytic

No jaundice or hepatosplenomegaly

Consider: Acute blood loss

Obstetric accident
Fetomaternal hemorrhage
Internal hemorrhage

Other

Galactosemia
Respiratory distress
Osteopetrosis
Leukemia

Jaundice generally present

Infections

Bacterial
Viral
Cytomegalic inclusion disease
Congenital syphilis
Congenital toxoplasmosis

From Oski, F. A. & Naiman, S. L., Haematologic problems of the newborn.
Vol. IV – Major problems in clinical Paediatrics. Consulting editor,
Schaffer, A. J., W. B. Saunders, Co., Philadelphia, 1966.

Note:

If citrate-anticoagulated whole blood is transfused rapidly hypocalcaemia will occur. If $\frac{1}{5}$ of the blood volume is infused in 10-15 mins, give 1ml of 10% calcium gluconate *slowly* for every 100ml of blood infused per 10 mins. This should be given into a different vein from the blood. Except in situations of liver impairment, if blood is being tranfused more slowly, then calcium need not be given.

(c) Platelets
   If a platelet transfusion is required, give 4-6 units/m^2
(d) Plasma
   Stored wet plasma is deficient in labile coagulation factors – particularly Factors V and VIII.
   Frozen plasma or fresh freeze dried plasma contains all coagulation factors.

Haemophilia

Frozen plasma or fresh freeze dried plasma can be used in emergencies to increase Factor VIII levels by up to about 20%. Fluid volume overloading requires that more concentrated products than normal be used for supportive therapy.

Cryoprecipitate: I.U. Factor VIII required =
$$\frac{\text{Wt in kg} \times \% \text{ Rise required}}{1.5}$$

1 bag/bottle contains 60-150 units depending on source and batch.

Minimum desired Factor VIII levels are shown below.

Haemarthrosis	15%
Mild trauma	15%
Dental extraction	30%
Minor surgery	30%
Multiple extractions	60%
Major surgery	60%
? Cerebral bleed	100%

For anything other than haemarthrosis or mild trauma a precise check on the Factor VIII level with a haematologist is indicated.

In general the treatment of haemophiliacs should preferably be performed by experienced practitioners only.

Oral Iron

Treatment 6mg/kg of elemental iron per day.
Give for 6-8 weeks.
For maintenance: Give 2mg/kg of the elemental iron per day.
BNF ferrous sulphate mixture: 12mg elemental iron/5ml;
ferrous gluconate (Fergon): 32mg elemental iron/5ml; ferrous
fumarate (Fersamal): 45mg elemental iron/5ml.
Check that adequate response to the iron therapy is obtained.
(1% per day rise in haematocrit)

Blood Pressure

Age	Normal Values	
Newborn	$^{85}/_{50}$	($\pm$ 10mm Hg)
6 months-1 year	$^{95}/_{65}$	($\pm$ 20mm Hg)
2-4 years	$^{100}/_{65}$	($\pm$ 20mm Hg)
5-10 years	$^{100}/_{55}$	($\pm$ 10mm Hg)
10 years +	$^{110}/_{60}$	($\pm$ 10mm Hg)

Infant Feeding

Requirements

Full term	Day	1	60ml/kg/day
		2	90ml/kg/day
		3	120ml/kg/day
		4	150ml/kg/day

Mean intake after first week is 160-170ml/kg/day
Preterm and small for gestational age infants may need up to
50% more than this.

Duration

Milk alone (either breast milk or 'modified' formulae) will
provide all the caloric requirements for the infant for the first
4-6 months.
Solid foods therefore need not be introduced before the age of
4 months.

Breast Feeding

This remains the best way of feeding a baby and all mothers
should be strongly encouraged to breast feed. However, the
mother's personal preference for either breast or bottle feeding
is of paramount importance. No mother who chooses to bottle
feed her infant should in any way be made to feel guilty or
inferior. The doctor's role is to explain the advantages of breast
feeding, to allow the mother to make her own decision and
then to ensure that whichever method is selected it is executed
correctly and that enjoyment is derived from it by both mother
and infant.
Breast feeding may commence any time after delivery –
approximately 6 hours at the latest.
Supplements of vitamin D (400 I.U./day) may be added after
1-2 weeks.
If the water supply is fluoridated to the extent of 1 part per
million then no additional supplementation is required.
Otherwise give infant 0.5mg/day.

Iron supplements do not seem necessary for full term healthy babies. If required, dose is 2mg/kg/day of elemental iron.
There are very few contraindications to breast feeding. Even extremely premature babies can be established on breast feeding when they are older provided mother has regularly expressed manually.

When it is *necessary* for the mother to receive any of the following medications she should not breast feed:

    (a) antithyroid drugs
    (b) antimetabolites
    (c) radioactive drugs
    (d) sulphonamides (if baby jaundiced)
    (e) tetracyclines
    (f) chloramphenicol
    (g) bromides

Many other drugs administered to the mother may be excreted in breast milk – usually in insignificant amounts. Information is not available on many new drugs.

Formula Feeding

There is a multiplicity of proprietary milks available. It is difficult to see significant differences between many of them, but on basic principles the modified milk formulae are to be preferred.

These include: Baby Milk Plus, Gold Cap SMA, Lactogen, Nan, Osterfeed, Ostermilk Complete, Premium SMA, Enfamil, Karitane Milk Food, Vitamilk 20, SMA.

Each packet carries instructions as to how the feed is to be made up. Milk is nearly always already fortified with iron and vitamins, so the infant's daily intake of these (as calculated from the packet) should be compared with his daily requirements (*see* below).

Special Formulae

Lactose intolerance:
    AL 110
    Galactomin 17
    Galactomin 18 (reduced fat)
    Glucose Nutramigen
    Prosobee
    Isomil

Cow's milk protein intolerance:
    Prosobee
    Soya food
    Isomil
Low sodium content:
    Edosol
    SMA Gold Cap
    Karitane Milk Food
    Enfamil
    SMA
    Vitamilk 20
Elemental diets:
    Flexical
    Pregestimil
    Vivonex

Dietary Requirements

Approximate daily dietary requirements of children under ordinary conditions

Age		3/12	6/12	9/12	1-3yrs	4-6yrs	7-9yrs
H_2O							
ml/kg		165	150	130	120	100	80
Energy							
MJ/kg		0.46	0.42	0.42	0.42	0.38	0.34
Protein							
g/kg		3.5	3.5	3.5	2.5	2.2	2.2
Minerals							
Ca	g	0.6	0.7	0.7	0.8	0.8	0.8
P	g	1.5	1.5	1.5	1.5	1.5	1.5
Fe	mg	6	7	8	8	10	12
Vitamins							
A	I.U	1500	1500	1500	2000	2500	3500
B1	mg	0.4	0.4	0.5	0.5	0.6	0.8
B2	mg	0.6	0.6	0.8	0.8	1.0	1.3
Niacin	mg	7	7	8	8	11	13
C	mg	35	35	35	40	40	40
D	I.U.	400	400	400	400	400	400

1 kcal = 4.2kJ

Meningitis

Infants and Children after the Neonatal Period

Pyogenic meningitis is a medical emergency and requires:
(a) Early diagnosis
(b) Specific high dosage antimicrobial therapy
(c) Intensive supportive care

Diagnosis

A high index of clinical suspension required. Lumbar puncture is mandatory for diagnosis. It is better to do too many lumbar punctures than to miss cases.

1. Lumbar Puncture
   Measure pressure and then send CSF for:
       chemistry – sugar
                       protein
       cell count and differential
       Gram stain
       countercurrent immunoelectrophoresis
       culture and sensitivity
       virus isolation
   If bloody tap, take three consecutive specimens and ask for differential cell count on each specimen.
   (Should be approx. 1 w.b.c. : 500-1000 r.b.c.)

Notes:

   (a) If CSF not clearing by the time the third specimen is taken and laboratory reports similar cell counts in all specimens – then consider possibility of:
       (i) intraventricular haemorrhage
       (ii) subarachnoid haemorrhage
   (b) Normal CSF values
       Pressure   40-200mm CSF
       Cells   Up to 5×10^6/l (0-5/mm^3)
       Protein   0.15-0.40g/l
       Sugar   2.5-4.5mmol/l (N$\frac{2}{3}$ blood sugar)
       Chloride   110-128mmol/l

In the neonate the protein and white cells can be significantly elevated in the first few days of life.

(c) If patient has been on antibiotics before admission, then CSF report may misleadingly suggest viral meningitis and there may be no growth. In such a case treat as for pyogenic meningitis.

2. Peripheral blood screen and ESR
3. Blood culture × 2
4. Electrolytes, sugar and urea
5. Chest X-ray
6. Urinalysis and culture
7. Swabs and needle aspiration of areas of focal sepsis
8. Acute and convalescent specimens for serology if aseptic meningitis. Specimens of pharyngeal washings, stool and urine usually also required for virus isolation.
9. Mantoux test – if tuberculous meningitis suspected.

Common Organisms Causing Pyogenic Meningitis

For practical purposes in children beyond the neonatal period there are three important micro-organisms responsible for pyogenic meningitis. In order of frequency these are:

1. *Haemophilus influenzae* type b:
    plemorphic Gram-negative coccobacilli
2. *Neisseria meningitidis*: Gram-negative diplococci
3. *Streptococcus pneumoniae*: Gram-positive diplococci

In the neonate *E. coli* is the commonest but this is rarely seen beyond about 6 weeks of age.

Specific Therapy

Antimicrobial therapy is commenced as soon as possible.

1. Initial therapy for all three common organisms: ampicillin 400mg/kg/24 hours i.v. 4 hourly. Administer ampicillin over 20 mins via drip chamber. Direct push should be avoided and slower infusions in dextrose containing solutions inadvisable and ineffective. In addition, chloramphenicol 100mg/kg/day i.v. in 4 divided doses, until the results of culture are known (addition of chloramphenicol necessary in view of isolation of *H. influenzae* type b resistant to ampicillin). When culture and sensitivity results are known, the less appropriate drug should be stopped.

2. Subsequent therapy depends on result of culture and sensitivity.
   (a) *H. influenzae* – ampicillin 400mg/kg/24 hours i.v. for 10-14 days in 6 divided doses
      or
      Chloramphenicol 100mg/kg/24 hours i.v. in 4 divided doses. After 48 hours decrease to 75mg/kg/day i.v. until substantial clinical improvement and patient drinking, then oral therapy to complete 10-14 day course.
   (b) *Streptococcus pneumoniae* and *N. meningitidis* – penicillin G 400mg/kg/24 hours i.v. in 6 divided doses for 10-14 days.

   Note:

   Dosage of penicillins must not be tapered with clinical improvement or changed to oral route.
   Chloramphenicol blood levels may be affected if patient is receiving phenobarbitone.

Allergy to Penicillin

A history of allergy to the penicillins needs careful evaluation in a child presenting with meningitis. True penicillin allergy is uncommon in childhood. Confusion may be caused by the transient exanthems associated with a wide variety of virus infections. If a definite history of penicillin allergy is obtained, rational decisions regarding alternative therapy can only be made with a knowledge of the sensitivities of organisms in the local community to the various antibacterial agents and in full consultation with a microbiologist. The following régime is suggested as a guide only.
1. Initial therapy for the three common organisms when patient allergic to penicillins:
      Chloramphenicol – 100mg/kg/day i.v. 6 hourly
      After 48 hours decrease to 75mg/kg/day
2. Subsequent therapy – after results of cultures available:
   (a) *H. influenzae* – chloramphenicol as above, i.v. until substantial clinical improvement and patient drinking then oral therapy to complete 10-14 day course.
   (b) *Streptococcus pneumoniae* – chloramphenicol as for *H. influenzae* and/or cefuroxime 100-150mg/kg/day i.v. 4 hourly.

Note:
This dose of cefuroxime exceeds the daily maximum
covered by the product licence at present.
Cephalosporins cross the blood brain barrier poorly
and in an irregular manner. If a decision is made to use
cefuroxime in the treatment of meningitis the minimal
inhibitory concentration (MIC) of the infecting
organism should be obtained as soon as possible and
blood and CSF levels of antibiotic should be monitored
regularly. Intrathecal cefuroxime cannot be
recommended at present.
Occasional cross-sensitisation between the penicillins
and the cephalosporins has been observed.

(c) *N. meningitidis* – chloramphenicol as for *H. influenzae*
or sulphadiazine 90mg/kg i.v. stat (max. 2g) and then
65mg/kg i.v. 4 hourly (max. 1g). Daily maximum is 6g.
Can change to oral route when substantial clinical
improvement and patient drinking. Orally give
300mg/kg/day in 4 doses to a maximum of 6g.

Neonatal Meningitis and Tuberculous Meningitis

Antimicrobial therapy – consult specific texts.

Partially Treated Meningitis

Prior antimicrobial therapy frequently sterilises the blood but
infrequently affects the ultimate isolation of a bacterial
pathogen from the CSF.
Initial therapy: ampicillin and chloramphenicol until culture
results available. If there is no growth on culture but clinical
picture and CSF are highly suggestive of purulent meningitis
then continue antibiotic treatment for 10-14 days.

Supportive Care

1. Nursing care
   Special nurse for infants, the semi-comatose, the convulsing
   or those in shock regardless of age.
   Monitor vital signs
   Control fever
   Maintain clear airway
   Administer drugs on schedule and care for vital i.v. line

2. Fever control
   Use of fans, sponging and antipyretics
3. Control of convulsions – *see* p.24
4. Fluids
   Initial i.v. rehydration if patient dehydrated; then maintenance fluids. Fluid restriction may become necessary in presence of cerebral oedema.

   Note:
   Do not overload patient or conversely render them hypovolaemic by inadequate initial hydration. Oral fluids when able to drink and reduce i.v. rate appropriately. Insert CVP line if hypotensive.

5. Cerebral oedema
   Treatment is controversial! Maintain clear airway and adequate oxygenation. Elevate head of bed. Do not overload with fluid, usually restrict to approx. $\frac{2}{3}$ normal requirement.
   May give:
   > mannitol 2g/kg/i.v. over 30-60 mins
   > dexamethasone 1.25mg/kg/i.v. stat
   > then 0.5mg/kg/day i.v. in 4 divided doses

   Alternative therapy includes intubation and barbiturate induced coma with artificial ventiltion in an intensive care unit.

Subsequent Care

1. Daily weight – increasing weight when calories and food are being restricted suggests inappropriate ADH secretion. Electrolytes and urine and serum osmolality required for diagnosis.
2. Daily head circumference.
3. Repeat peripheral w.b.c. and ESR twice weekly.
4. Stopping therapy: at end of treatment period review clinical state of child, temperature chart, w.b.c. and ESR. Repeat lumbar puncture recommended by many to ensure CSF sterile, w.b.c. less than $50/mm^3$, sugar and protein near normal.
   Observe child for 48 hours after stopping antimicrobial therapy and if clinically well discharge.

Notes:

1. Persistent fever – consider:
   (a) Continuing CNS infection
   (b) Brain abscess
   (c) Subdural abscess
   (d) Infection elsewhere
   (e) Thrombophlebitis following i.v. infusion
   (f) Dehydration
   (g) Unknown cause but settles when therapy finished
2. Drug fever:
   Rash may appear. Child develops fever approximately 7 days after onset of treatment. Particularly with high dose ampicillin.
3. Intrathecal antibiotics:
   Controversial. Most authorities do not recommend it. In neonatal meningitis where ventriculitis suspected the placement of a ventricular reservoir is the established means of delivering antibiotic. 1-2mg of gentamicin daily increasing if necessary to 5-8mg. Continue until smears negative and no growth on culture on 3 consecutive days. Intrathecal therapy usually necessary for staphylococcal meningitis as cloxacillin and cephalosporins penetrate CSF poorly.
4. Prophylaxis of contacts:
   This issue is controversial.
   For close contacts of patients with *N. meningitidis* infection, some would recommend giving sulphadiazine for 5 days, providing the organism is sensitive. Alternatives are rifampicin or a tetracycline.
   If *H. influenzae* or *Streptococcus pneumoniae* is isolated, prophylaxis is not usually recommended though close contacts of the case should be under medical review if they develop symptoms.

Poisoning

General

1. If contacted by phone, advise induction of vomiting by stimulating back of throat.
   Except
   (i) If child is semiconscious or convulsing
   (ii) If child has ingested:
        acid, alkali, petrol, or kerosene
   In hospital, vomiting can be induced by giving the child syrup of ipecac orally in the following dose:
       1 year – 15ml
       2 yrs   – 20ml
       3 yrs   – 25ml
       > 3 yrs – 30ml

FOLLOWED BY APPROX. 200ml OF WATER or CORDIAL, as syrup of ipecac may fail to work on an otherwise empty stomach. Do not give milk with syrup of ipecac. If vomiting has not occurred within 15 minutes, the dose may be repeated once. It is important that the fluid extract of ipecac is NOT used as it is a much more potent solution, and serious, even fatal, side effects may follow its ingestion. It has been shown that induced vomiting with ipecac brings about a more complete removal of stomach contents than does stomach washout, but in certain situations the latter is to be preferred:
   (i) If the child is semiconscious on arrival – the level of consciousness may deteriorate further while waiting for the child to vomit, and the resulting risk of aspiration of vomitus into the lungs is high.
   (ii) If the child has ingested a tricyclic antidepressant coma may develop very rapidly and the same complication as described above can occur.
   (iii) If the child has ingested an anti-emetic.

If the child is unconscious or has ingested petroleum products then a cuffed endotracheal tube must be in place before stomach washout is attempted.
Following ingestion of corrosives, neither induction of vomiting nor stomach washout should be performed.
All vomitus should be saved for analysis of the substance ingested.

2. Except where a specific oral antidote is available, activated charcoal should be given after the stomach has been cleared.
   If a stomach tube has been passed, then following the washout a cupful of activated charcoal of soupy consistency (1-2 tablespoons in 2.5ml H_2O) should be left in the stomach. If vomiting has been induced then the child should be encouraged to drink this solution; though as the child is likely to be fairly unco-operative by this stage, a lengthy period should not be spent on persuasion.
3. Surface poisons: Copious water irrigation. Do not apply specific antidotes to skin.

CORROSIVES (ACIDS & ALKALIS)

Clinically
1. Burns of lips, mouth, tongue and pharynx may be seen.
2. Drooling from mouth.
3. Respiratory distress may indicate laryngeal burns and need for tracheostomy.
4. Substernal burning and epigastric pain.
   Vomiting (possibly blood or sloughed mucosa).
   Diarrhoea
5. Shock.
6. Oesophageal and stomach perforation.
7. Early stricture may occur.

Management
1. Rinse mouth and pharynx with copious water.
   Milk may be used for acid burns and fruit juice for alkali burns.
2. If child able to swallow saliva start feeding with clear fluids and progress as tolerated to normal diet.

For more severe burns:
3. Morphine 0.2mg/kg/dose
4. Benzyl penicillin i.m. or i.v. (dose for age).
5. If unable to swallow, then i.v. fluids (*see* p.48).
6. Oesophagoscopy if not in shock. This should be performed 12-24 hours after ingestion to assess damage.

If no abnormality detected, or only patchy oedema of intact mucosa seen, then no treatment is required and the child is allowed home once normal feeding is restored.

If areas of white mucosal slough are seen, these should be regarded as potential strictures and mangement is as follows:

(a) Penicillin V and cloxacillin in dose for age for 2 weeks.
(b) Prednisone 3-5mg/kg/day – at least until repeat oesophagoscopy.
(c) Ba swallow on tenth day and assess progress by repeat examinations at about 10-day intervals so long as lesion progresses.
(d) Oesophagoscopy may be repeated at 3 weeks if indicated.
(e) Bougienage may be required for developing stricture.

IRON POISONING

MAY BE FATAL IN DOSES AS LOW AS 40mg/kg ELEMENTAL IRON

Ferrous sulphate – 200mg tab contains 60mg elemental iron
BNF ferrous sulphate mixture – 12mg elemental iron/5ml
Ferrous gluconate – 300mg tab contains 35mg elemental iron
Ferrous gluconate – 32mg elemental iron/5ml
Ferrous fumarate – 200mg tab contains 65mg elemental iron
Ferrous fumarate – 45mg elemental iron/5ml

Phases of Intoxication

1. Haemorrhagic gastroenteritis within a few hours of ingestion.
2. Delayed shock 1-2 days after ingestion.
3. Liver necrosis
4. Obstruction from post-necrotic scarring 1-2 months later.

Management

1. Emesis
2. Lavage with $NaHCO_3$ solution
   (3-4 tablespoons $NaHCO_3$ to 1 litre H_2O)

3. Leave 5-10g desferrioxamine in stomach
4. X-ray abdomen – portable in ward
5. Serum iron
6. Enema
7. Desferrioxamine 20mg/kg/i.m. stat and subsequent doses of 20mg/kg/i.m. 4 hourly depending on clinical response. If patient is severely shocked, ensure adequate renal function before giving desferrioxamine. If poisoning very severe may require to be given i.v., though i.m. route to be used as soon as possible; i.v. dose not to exceed 15mg/kg/hr *or* 100mg/kg/24 hours.

LEAD POISONING

Investigations

Urine:
  porphyrins
  lead
  aminoacids
  glucose
  blood
X-ray:
  abdomen
  wrists and knees
Serum lead
Blood screen
Liver function tests
Electrolytes and urea

Management

1. If acute poisoning:
     emesis or lavage
     give cup of H_2O containing 30g sodium sulphate.

Note:
If lead present in intestines give a stat dose of dimercaprol (BAL) 3mg/kg/i.m. (10% solution contains 100mg/ml)

2. If chronic poisoning:
   (a) Without encephalopathy
       (i) Calcium disodium versenate (200mg/ml) 30mg/kg
           diluted to a 0.2-0.4% solution with 5% dextrose, i.v.
           over 1-2 hours.
           Repeat twice daily. May be given over 5 days;
           interval of 2 days before repeat course.
       (ii) Lead colic:
           10ml of 10% Ca gluconate i.v. VERY SLOWLY.
           Repeat PRN. May also use antispasmodics, e.g.
           atropine, 0.01mg/kg/dose (max. 0.4mg). Repeat 4-6
           hourly.
       (iii) For long-term oral deleading:
           N-acetyl-D, L-penicillamine 30-40mg/kg/day in 2
           or 3 divided doses in fruit juice between meals.
   (b) With encephalopathy
       (i) Avoid fluid overload, so calcium disodium
           versenate may require to be given i.m. –
           60mg/kg/day in divided doses with local
           anaesthetic.
       (ii) Cerebral oedema:
           Mannitol 2g/kg given as 20% solution over 30-60
           min. i.v.
           Dexamethasone (*see* drug index)
           May require neurosurgical intervention
       (iii) Convulsions:
           Paraldehyde 0.15ml/kg/dose i.m.

PETROLEUM DISTILLATES

Includes: kerosene, paint thinner, and turpentine. Ingestion of
more than 10ml may be fatal.

Management

1. DO NOT INDUCE VOMITING.
2. Gastric lavage ONLY if cuffed endotracheal tube in place. It
   may be helpful, in determining the amount of petroleum
   distillate ingested, to take an erect X-ray of the abdomen
   after the child has drunk a glass of water. If a double fluid

level is seen, this suggests that a significant volume of distillate has been ingested and is still in the stomach.

3. Following lavage, leave 30g of sodium sulphate dissolved in 1 cup of H_2O in stomach.
4. Baseline chest X-ray.
5. No prophylactic antibiotic.
6. Continuing observations
    – Respiratory system:
        Pulmonary oedema – *see* p.7
        Pneumonitis – humidified O_2; prednisone 5mg/kg/day
        Bacterial infection – penicillin ± cloxacillin in dose for age
    – CNS:
    Severe cases may show signs of CNS depression and irritation.

PHENOTHIAZINES

Particularly: prochlorperazine (Stemetil), trifluoperazine (Stelazine), and perphenazine (Fentazin), produce drowsiness and extrapyramidal symptoms.

Management

1. Gastric lavage
2. Activated charcoal　} *see* introduction to poisons
3. Observations:
    Respiratory rate
    Pulse
    BP
    CNS
4. If evidence of extrapyramidal symptoms:
    Diphenhydramine hydrochloride (Benadryl) – 0.5-1mg/ kg/dose i.v.
    or
    Benztropine mesylate (Cogentin) – 0.5-1mg i.v.
    To prevent development of extrapyramidal symptoms Benadryl may be used i.m. or orally in a dose of 5mg/kg/24 hours divided q.i.d.

Note:

Cardiovascular complications discussed under tricyclic

antidepressants (p.95) may also occur with phenothiazine overdose.

SALICYLATES

Aspirin
Methyl salicylate (Oil of Wintergreen)
  1 tsp. = 2.7g salicylate

Clinical impression of severity of more importance than blood salicylate level as latter is dependent upon several factors. However, the nomogram based on blood salicylate level may

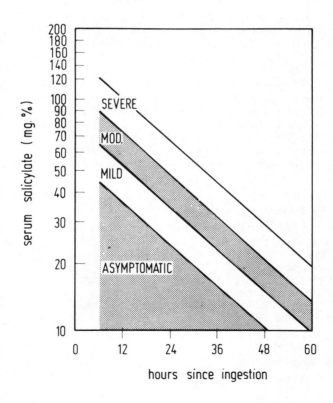

be of some use if predicting severity, provided it is remembered that it cannot be applied:
 (i) Until an adequate period has been allowed for absorption of most of drug – for practical purposes this is taken as 6 hours
(ii) If intoxication has occurred after repeated doses over a period of time. Thus it is only of use with patients who have ingested salicylate in a single dose.

Generally patients show signs of intoxication at lower serum salicylate levels when poisoning has occurred after repeated doses over a period of time.

Effects

1. Increased pulmonary ventilation → respiratory alkalosis → loss of HCO_3^- in urine to compensate.
2. Increased metabolic rate AND disturbed metabolism of carbohydrates leading to increased production of organic acids.
   This plus the loss of HCO_3^-, causes a metabolic acidosis.

Generally speaking, children under the age of 4 are rarely alkalotic and often have a metabolic acidosis. The disruption of CHO metabolism is also responsible for the changes in blood sugar which may be found. In some cases hyperglycaemia with glycosuria may occur. In others hypoglycaemia may develop and will require therapy.

Symptoms and Signs

Hyperventilation – more increase in depth than rate of respiration.
Fever
Sweating
Dehydration – from fever, sweating, hyperventilation.
Haemorrhagic tendencies
CNS signs – restlessness; delirium; hallucinations; coma; convulsions.

Investigations

Blood sugar

Electrolytes and urea
Capillary blood gases
Serum salicylate level
Urine – positive test for reducing substances AFTER boiling
urine confirms presence of salicylates.

Observations

Respiratory rate
Temperature
Pulse
CNS
pH of each urine specimen passed

Monitor

Electrolytes and urea ⎫
Capillary pH ⎬ 6-hourly initially
P_{CO_2} ⎭

Therapy

1. Induce emesis if ingestion has occurred within last 6 hours.
2. Activated charcoal (*see* p.86).
3. Tepid sponging if hyperpyrexic.
4. Vit K_1 5-10 mg i.m.
5. If child under 2, or at any age shows evidence of
   intoxication other than simple hyperventilation, then i.v.
   fluids should be given.

   0.18% NaCl + 4% dextrose

   20ml/kg in first hour, and thereafter as calculated,
   depending on state of hydration of patient, using section on
   electrolyte therapy. Add potassium 3mmol/kg/day to
   solution as soon as urine output is established. In presence
   of overt shock on presentation, commence with plasma or
   0.9% NaCl (whichever is most readily available) at rate of
   20ml/kg given over 1 hour and then continue as above.
   Continue i.v. fluids until dehydration is corrected and child
   is showing signs of symptomatic improvement.

Place of Bicarbonate

In any child under age of 4 who is receiving i.v. therapy.
In any child who is shown from blood gases to be acidaemic.

Aim of Bicarbonate

To maintain blood pH within normal range because toxic effects of salicylate are more marked in acidaemic patients. To maintain pH of urine greater than 7.0 because excretion of salicylate is increased in alkaline urine.

Method

Give 3mmol/kg of $NaHCO_3$ i.v. stat. Plus additional 30mmol of $NaHCO_3$ per litre solution initially, and thereafter adjust as necessary depending on blood pH and pH of urine.
If severe acidaemia persists despite addition of above, supplements of HCO_3^- can be given in doses of 3mmol/kg i.v. over 5 minutes and repeated twice at 10 minute intervals if required.

Other Complications

Occasionally in severely affected cases other complications may arise:

    Acute pulmonary oedema (p.7)
    Congestive heart failure (p.9)
    Convulsions (p.24)
    Tetany – calcium gluconate 10% (100mg/ml) 100mg/kg
    bodyweight infused SLOWLY i.v.

Consider dialysis – extracorporeal or peritoneal – if:

 (i) patient cannot be treated with large volumes of fluid
 (ii) there is lack of response to HCO_3^- therapy
(iii) patient in coma or having seizures

If respiratory depression occurs then the patient will require assisted ventilation to ensure continued removal of CO_2.

TRICYCLIC ANTIDEPRESSANTS

Includes:
amitriptyline
imipramine
nortriptyline
trimipramine
protriptyline
desipramine

Serious toxic effects should be expected if ingested dose is more than 20mg/kg.

Clinical Features

Brought about by combination of powerful anticholinergic effects, and less marked sympathomimetic effects; in cases where large doses have been ingested, the drugs appear also to exert a direct toxic effect on the myocardium and conducting tissue of the heart.

Mild – Moderate

Some depression of level of consciousness, possibly alternating with periods of agitation.

Ataxia ± nystagmus

Signs of anticholinergic effects:
tachycardia
dry mouth
thirst
bladder distension
decreased bowel sounds
dilated pupils

Severe

CNS:
coma
widely dilated pupils – unreactive to light.
hypertonicity; muscular twitchings; convulsions.
respiratory depression

CVS:
ECG abnormal – prolonged P-R interval; widening of QRS;

S-T segment depression; T wave flattening; prominent
U wave

arrhythmias – bradycardia; supraventricular tachycardia;
ventricular extrasystoles and tachycardia; ventricular
fibrillation; LBBB; AV block
hypotension
myocarditis
cardiac arrest

Metabolic acidosis with hypokalaemia.
Sudden death up to 96 hours after ingestion.

Note:

Evidence of recovery usually seen 18-24 hours after ingestion.
Before this time the finding of fixed, widely dilated pupils in a
comatose patient cannot be interpreted in its usual poor
prognostic fashion.

Management

1. If patient conscious when seen, induce vomiting by tickling
   back of throat. Do not use syrup of ipecac (*see* p.85).
   If level of conscious is impaired, wash out stomach only
   when cuffed endotracheal tube is in place. Lavage only of
   benefit if seen within 3 hours of ingestion as absorption
   from GI tract is rapid.
2. Give cupful of activated charcoal or leave some in stomach
   after lavage (*see* p.86).
3. ADMIT ALL CASES TO MEDICAL ICU FOR MONITORING FOR
   4 DAYS.
4. Observations
   Respiratory rate
   Pulse
   BP
   Level of consciousness
   Input – output chart
   ECG
5. Forced diuresis or dialysis of no benefit in increasing rate of
   removal of drug. In fact excess i.v. fluids may worsen
   cardiac state.
6. Convulsions
   When muscular twitchings are seen, treatment should be

given as convulsions are likely to follow.

Use   i.m. paraldehyde 0.15ml/kg/dose

or   i.v. diazepam (Valium) (*see* p.24)

7. Respiratory depression. If rate or depth of respiration falls, then artificial ventilation may be necessary. (*see* p.116).

8. i.v. sodium bicarbonate and i.v. potassium according to laboratory results.

9. Anticholinergic effects may be counteracted by neostigmine 0.25-1mg i.v. Repeated as necessary.

10. CVS
   (a) Arrhythmias:
      (i) Supraventricular arrhythmias. May respond to neostigmine 0.25-1mg i.v. Also try propranolol 0.2mg/kg/i.m.
      (ii) Ventricular extrasystoles and tachycardia. Lignocaine. Initially 1-4mg/kg/i.v stat. Then continuous infusion of 10-40μg/kg/min. Make up solution as 5% dextrose. d.c. countershock for unresponsive VT.
      (iii) Ventricular fibrillation (*see* p.8).
      (iv) Heart block and bradycardia – i.v. pacing if of haemodynamic significance.
   (b) Cardiac failure:
      Digitalise i.v. (*see* p.9)
      Frusemide (Lasix) 1-5mg/kg/i.v.
      Glucagon 50μg/kg/i.v. every 30 mins. as required.
   (c) Hypotension:
      Management is difficult and will depend on associated features, e.g. presence or absence of arrhythmias. If available, a cardiologist should be consulted. Treat as for cardiac failure (*see above*). If no improvement then:
      (i) Isoprenaline
         1mg in 250ml of 5% dextrose. Give 0.5-1ml/min i.v. under ECG control and titrate against effect. Stop if heart rate > 200/min.
      (ii) Adrenaline 0.25-1.0mg/kg/min i.v. Titrate against effect.
      (iii) Volume replacement – as judged by wedge pressure. Measurement (Swan-Ganz catheter). Infuse to mean wedge pressure of 15mmHg. This is preferable to CVP measurement, but if unavailable use CVP as guideline.

Notes:

1. Arrhythmias may develop during (i) and (ii)
2. Monitor response to therapy according to peripheral state, urine output (*see* p.5) and blood pressure. Blood pressure is the least important of the three.

Renal Problems

ACUTE UNCOMPLICATED NEPHRITIS

Investigations
1. Throat swab
2. β_1 C globulin
3. Blood screen and ESR
4. Electrolytes and urea
5. Microscopy of urine cells and casts
6. MSU for culture and sensitivities
7. ASO titre (and if ASO negative, especially with a skin
   primary: antistreptokinase, antihyaluronidase,
   antistreptococcal deoxyfibonuclease B)

Observations
1. Input-output chart
2. Regular BP – 4 hourly
3. Daily weight

Therapy
1. Bed rest and fluid balance for at least 24 hours.
2. Penicillin V (dose for age) – 10 days.
   No need for subsequent prophylactic penicillin – second
   attacks very uncommon.

Course
In the absence of any complications, prolonged bed rest and
hospitalisation are unnecessary. However, apart from mild
cases, all these children should be admitted for initial
investigation and observation.

Notes:
1. Persistence of microscopic haematuria:

0-3 months	50%
3-6 months	30%
1 year	10%

2. Duration of elevated ESR:

0-3 months	50%
3-6 months	25%
Over 1 year	0%

COMPLICATIONS OF ACUTE NEPHRITIS
(For treatment of Acute Renal Failure – *see* p.104)

1. Hypertension

Mild – reserpine 0.01-0.04mg/kg in single dose
i.m. ± hydrallazine (Apresoline) 0.1mg/kg i.m.

Severe – diazoxide 5mg/kg rapidly i.v. (effect may last up to 48 hours)
or reserpine 0.07mg/kg/dose i.m.
+ hydrallazine 0.1-0.2mg/kg/dose i.v. Repeat in 6-12 hours. Dose of hydrallazine may be progressively increased, according to response to 1mg/kg/dose

2. High Blood Urea

(a) Restrict protein to 0.3-0.5g/kg/day or nil for 3-4 days. High CHO intake to provide calories – $4.2mJ/m^2$. (4.2 megajoules = 1000 Cal)

(b) Fluids – urine output + $300ml/m^2/day$

(c) Daily electrolytes and urea – observe for raised K^+.

3. Post-oliguric Phase of Diuresis

Can develop electrolyte imbalances – daily check of electroytes and urea.

COMPARISON OF TYPICAL CASES OF NEPHROSIS & NEPHRITIS

		Nephritis	**Nephrosis**
Aetiology		Post ß haem. strep.	Idiopathic ? postviral
Age		Rare less than 3 5-15 years	3-10 years Maximum around 3 years
Presentation		Haematuria	Oedema
Clinical Onset		Sudden	Gradual
Oedema		±	+ + +
Temperature		↑	Normal
B.P.		Normal or ↑	Normal
Urine	blood	+ +	–
	casts	red cell	Hyaline; fatty
	Protein	$< 60mg/m^2/day$	$> 60mg/m^2/day$
Blood	ASOT ß$_1$ C	↑	Normal
	globulin(C$_3$)	↑	Normal
	cholesterol	Normal	↑
Plasma protein electrophoresis		Normal alb:glob ratio	Reversal of alb:glob ratio (hypoalbuminaemia)

NEPHROTIC SYNDROME

Therapy of 'Typical' Case

i.e. – age group 3-10; no haematuria; no complications; no hypertension

1. Initial Investigations:

   Height, weight and surface area

   Urine:

   MSU for culture and sensitivity

   Microscopy (should be done by house physician on the ward)

   Creatinine clearance (an accurately timed urine collection is required: 12-24 hours. Send also blood for serum creatinine)

Blood:
  Electrolytes and urea
  Blood screen and ESR
  Serum cholesterol
  P. protein electrophoresis
  β_1 C globulin (C_3). Also C_4.
Others:
  Heaf test (pre-steroid check)
  Chest X-ray
  Plain X-ray abdomen – for renal outlines

2. Continuing observations:
   (a) Watch closely for signs of infection e.g. pneumococcal peritonitis can occur
   (b) Regular blood pressure if haematuria
   (c) Daily weight
   (d) Daily ward testing of urine for protein
   (e) 24-hour urine for protein twice weekly

3. Prednisone:
   60 mg/m^2 to max. of 100mg per day (in 3 divided doses) until urine free of protein for 5 days.
   Then continue steroid therapy in gradually reducing dosage over a 2-5 monthly period, giving daily, alternate days, or three days per week.
   If relapse occurs, start again from beginning.

4. Indications for a renal biopsy:
   (a) Unusual presentation –
          e.g. greater than 10 years old
          haematuria
          raised blood pressure
   (b) After second relapse on steroids.
   (c) No response to steroids.

5. Other therapy
   (a) Diuretics – use if:
        (i) Patient very uncomfortable due to oedema on presentation
        (ii) Prior to biopsy on oedematous patient
             frusemide (Lasix) 2mg/kg/stat. i.m.
             and
             2-5mg/kg/day orally if necessary.
             spironolactone 5mg/kg/day.
   (b) Cytotoxic agents – consider in:
        (i) Steroid-dependent cases with major side effects –
             e.g. growth retardation
             osteoporosis

    labile BP
    diabetes mellitus
(ii) If non-steroid responsive and biopsy suggests
    membrano-proliferative
        or
    focal sclerosing glomerular nephritis

Cyclosphosphamide:
3mg/kg/day maximum 6-8 weeks.
If possible, induce steroid remission, then administer
cyclophosphamide while continuing to give steroids in a
dose which, from previous experience with the patient,
has been sufficient to maintain remission. Upon
completion of course of cyclophosphamide, begin to
decrease steroids weekly to zero by 8 weeks. Monitor
while cell count – no need to induce leucopenia.
Side effects:
    haemorrhagic cystitis
    bone marrow depression
    alopecia
    ?sterility

Note:
General points regarding use of cytotoxic agents in this
condition –
(a) Cytotoxic drugs should not be used to induce initial
    remission.
(b) Decision to use them must not be taken lightly
    especially in view of reported sterility and potential
    carcinogenisis.
(c) The position, side effects, etc. must be discussed
    with parents before embarking upon therapy.

RENAL BIOPSY

Preparation
1. Plain film of abdomen with lead marker over right kidney
   (in right renal angle) (± tomogram).
2. If suggestion of any abnormality in plain film – IVP
3. Coagulation studies.
4. Group and cross-match 1 unit of blood.

5. Premed:
> Nil orally for 4 hours prior to biopsy
> Consult the person performing the biopsy for premed.

Contra-indications

Absolute:
> bleeding diathesis
> severe hypertension

Relative:
> solitary kidney
> abnormal renal position
> cystic changes suggestive of hydronephrosis
> UTI

Post-Biopsy Care

BP, pulse and respiration at 3-minute invervals for 20 minutes; bed rest for 24 hours; encourage oral fluids.

The persistence of haematuria for more than 24 hours may be significant, and should be brought to the attention of the person who performed the biopsy.

TREATMENT OF ACUTE RENAL FAILURE DUE TO 'RENAL CAUSES'

1. **Oliguria**

> Defined as less than $250ml/m^2/day$
> To differentiate oliguria due to inadequate fluid replacement *see* p.5
> Total daily fluid:
> $300ml/m^2$ + urine output + other losses
> i.v. as 10-20% dextrose
> Orally:
> > no proteins
> > high carbohydrate/fat
> > low potassium
> > can add caloreen powder

2. Hyperkalaemia

Medical emergency if K^+ greater than 8mmol/l.
ECG changes: peaked T waves, widening QRS,
arrhythmias, prolonged PR, or absent P waves.

(a) Calcium gluconate
10% solution, 0.5ml/kg i.v. over 2-4 mins under ECG
control

then

(b) $NaHCO_3$ 2.5mmol/kg i.v.
or Glucose and soluble insulin: 1ml/kg 50% glucose
(0.5g/ml) plus 1 unit insulin/4g glucose.
or Resonium A
5g daily orally in 4 divided doses.
Mix with milk and honey to enhance palatability.
Estimated that 1g resin exchanges 2.8-3.5mmol of K^+
or Dialysis

Duration of Action of Measures used for Hyperkalaemia

	Onset	Duration
Calcium gluconate	few mins	30-60 mins
$NaCHO_3$	few mins	1-2 hours
Insulin glucose	few mins	2-4 hours
Resins	$\frac{1}{2}$ hour	3-4 hours

3. Hypertension

Diazoxide – 5mg/kg rapidly i.v. Effect usually lasts 3-4
hours but may persist up to 48 hours.

4. Seizures

see Treatment of Convulsions (p.24)

5. Other Complications which are Indications for Dialysis

(a) Fluid overload
(b) Water intoxication with hyponatraemia; altered
consciousness; or convulsions

    (c) Hyperkalaemia
    (d) Haemorrhagic diathesis
    (e) Deterioration in clinical state
    (f) Severe uraemia or rapidly rising urea – more than
        50mmol/l (300mg/100ml)

Monitor

1. Level of consciousness
2. Weight
3. Electrolytes
4. ECG
5. Haemoglobin, platelets
6. BP
7. Ca^{++} and $PO_4^{=}$

URINARY TRACT INFECTION

Consider in all cases of:
    Pyrexia
    Febrile convulsions
    Failure to thrive
    Vomiting/diarrhoea
    Abdominal pain
    Past history of UTI
    Enuresis
    Abnormality of bladder function, e.g. neurogenic bladder,
    spina bifida
    Unexplained neonatal jaundice

Diagnosis

1. Urine for culture and sensitivity and cell count.
   Gram stain if urine obtained by suprapubic aspiration.
   All urines should be stored at 4°C prior to transportation
   for culture.

   Techniques of collection:
   (a) Bag specimen. Commonly used but only reliable for

screening. If $> 10\ 000$ organisms/ml ($10 \times 10^6/l$) then consider repeating or performing suprapubic aspiration.

(b) Clean catch specimen. More reliable but definitive diagnosis requires 2 consecutive specimens with $> 100\ 000$ organisms/ml ($100 \times 10^6/l$).

(c) Suprapubic aspiration. This technique should be carried out in acutely ill patients in whom an urgent diagnosis is required, or when there is any doubt over bag or clean catch specimens. See below for technique.

Pyuria:

> 10 w.b.c. per mm^3 ($10^6/l$) suggests inflammation in the genito-urinary tract. It does not necessarily mean that there is urinary tract infection as white cells in the urine can be found in such conditions as vulvo-vaginitis, trauma, foreign body, glomerulonephritis etc. It may support the diagnosis of a urinary tract infection where there has been prior antibiotic therapy. Pyuria may be absent in some patients who have persistent or recurrent bouts of infection.

2. Blood screen – w.b.c. and differential, ESR.

Management

1. Accurate diagnosis
2. Chemotherapy
   (a) Duration – 5 days (longer therapy may be indicated if underlying structural abnormality is suspected)
   (b) If possible await sensitivity, otherwise treat with:
       (i) sulphonamide
          or
       (ii) co-trimoxazole
          or
       (iii) amoxycillin
          see Pharmacopoeia for dosages
   (c) Repeat urine examination 24 hours after termination of therapy
3. Document: height and weight; BP; urea and electrolytes
4. Investigation – either immediately after assured diagnosis, or $^4/_{52}$ after urine clears, obtain IVP and possibly a micturating cystourethrogram.
   Request consultation with genito-urinary surgeon if anatomical abnormality found.

Note:

Treat asymptomatic bacteruria only if confirmed by bladder tap.

Technique for suprapubic bladder puncture

Preparation:

Give the infant a substantial amount of fluid to drink about half an hour before procedure.
Sedate an older child if apprehensive.
Postpone attempt if child passes urine within preceding half hour.

Procedure:

Place infant on a firm surface in a supine frog position (*see* Fig a). Assistant should hold legs with her hands and steady the body with her elbows.
The bladder is percussed to ensure it is full, and the skin between the umbilicus and symphysis pubis cleaned with a suitable antiseptic. Local anaesthetic is not usually required. Using a 3.8cm (1½in) 22 gauge needle attached to a 5ml sterile syringe, puncture skin in the midline 1-2cm above the symphyisis and pass the needle quickly down at an angle of 45-60° until the bladder is penetrated to a depth of about 2-3cm (*see* Fig. b).
Aspirate urine gently, withdraw the needle and seal it with a sterile cork.

Note:

Ensure the bladder is full before attempting this procedure. Unsuccessful attempts at bladder puncture needlessly frighten the child, especially one who may need repeated examinations.

A word of caution. Frequently the baby 'beats you' by micturating just as you are about to proceed. To avoid this:
1. Make sure you have everything ready to hand before you start to undress the child.
2. Ask your assistant to clamp the penis or hold the vulva together between finger and thumb until you have actually entered the bladder.

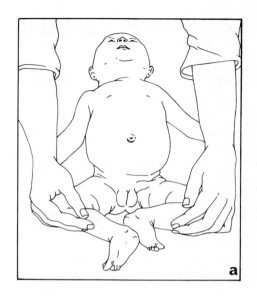

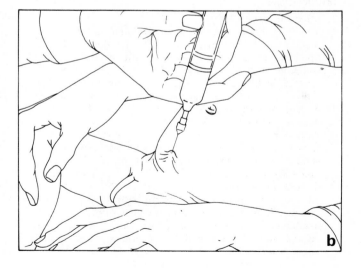

Respiratory Problems

ASTHMA/WHEEZY BRONCHITIS

Assess Severity

1. History – duration of attack; rate of deterioration.
2. Clinical examination – assess chest shape as evidence of chronic airway obstruction.

   Note:
   Beware especially of those children with hyperinflated and silent chests (poor air entry with minimal wheeze). They have severe airway obstruction.

3. Consider blood gas analysis. (*see* below)

Investigations

1. Microbiology
   The majority of acute attacks of asthma in childhood are precipitated by respiratory tract infection due to viruses. Such attacks of asthma associated with infection are sometimes called wheezy bronchitis, but there seems little purpose in differentiating the two conditions in that individual attacks are indistinguishable clinically, and the management of both is similar. Bronchitis without wheezing is a separate entity.
   Although the majority of infections are due to viruses, superadded bacterial infection of the lower respiratory tract should be considered and appropriate bacterial cultures taken. Nose and throat swabs for bacterial culture are of limited value in lower respiratory tract infections. Blood cultures taken prior to starting antibiotic therapy are more reliable. Sputum specimens, or tracheal aspirates, if available, should be sent for culture and sensitivities. Virus cultures should be taken in those centres where there are appropriate facilities.
2. Blood screen with differential w.b.c.
3. Chest X-ray – on first admission and in the seriously ill

child, but may not be needed for the mild asthmatic attack
with frequent previous admissions.

4. Arterial blood gases: indications essentially clinical and
   only *after* resuscitative measures.
   (a) If child remains very unwell (e.g. cyanosed) 30 minutes
       after hospital therapy begun.
   (b) If condition deteriorates markedly during hospital stay.
   (c) Repeat after 1 hour if child not markedly improved and
       original figures significantly abnormal
       e.g. $Pa\text{CO}_2$ 6.67kPa (50mm Hg) or less
              $Pa\text{CO}_2$ 6.00kPa (45mm Hg) or more
   (d) Further blood gases should be taken hourly or even
       more frequently as indicated. An indwelling arterial
       catheter may be required.
   (e) Marginal blood gas values are of greater significance in
       a tiring child.

Immediate Therapy

Before giving any drugs, obtain history of previous medication,
past and present, noting particularly any unusual reactions.
Many patients have received large doses of theophylline and
sympathomimetics before admission and great care should be
exercised. Drug therapy should follow an additive sequence
depending on the initial severity of the attack and response to
treatment.

Note:
If child less than six months then 1, 2 and 4 do not apply.
See under 'other therapy' below for initial management of a
young infant. If condition does not improve with these
measures some would give steroids in dose outlined under 3
below.

1. Sympathomimetics
   (a) By inhalation: salbutamol solution via nebulizer driven
       by pump or air/O_2 cylinder at 8l/min. Salbutamol
       solution (5mg/ml) in dosage 0.15mg/kg diluted to 2ml
       volume in normal saline. Repeat 4-6 hourly.
   (b) By parental injection (if too dyspnoeic to manage
       inhalation or unco-operative):
       (i) Adrenaline 0.1ml/min of 1:1000 s.c. until spasm
           ceases, or to maximum of 0.75ml. Administer via
           insulin syringe.
           Stop if nausea/vomiting occurs or pulse rate rises to

30/min. over initial level.
or
(ii) Ethylnoradrenaline (2mg/ml) i.m. according to age
and size. Rough guide:

1-2 years	0.3ml
3-4 years	0.5ml
5-6 years	0.7ml
7+years	1.0ml

2. Aminophylline

If in spite of measures indicated under 1. there is insufficient
relief after 10-15 minutes, set up i.v. line.

Loading dose of aminophylline 5mg/kg SLOWLY over 15-30
minutes.

Look for: restlessness, irritability, vomiting.

Ask for: nausea, peculiar taste (as of copper) in mouth.

If any of these occur – stop.

Then continuous infusion of 0.9mg/kg/hour.

Note:

No loading dose should be given if child has been on a
regular Theophylline-containing medication.

3. Steroids

Steroid therapy should be considered if the child has had a
course of steroids in the previous 6 months, if the child is
gravely ill on admission, or if child not markedly improved
30 minutes after aminophylline begun. Steroids will not
produce immediate benefit and other measures will need to
be taken.

Hydrocortisone hemisuccinate 4mg/kg 2 hourly i.v.

4. Salbutamol intravenously

If child is still severely wheezy after another 2 hours, or
earlier if sympathomimetics have not been administered.
Give 8μg/kg as bolus slowly over 5 minutes then
8μg/kg/hour as continuous infusion.

Note:

There is very little experience with i.v. salbutamol in
children. It should only be given to a child on a cardiac
monitor in an intensive care unit.

Other Therapy

1. Oxygen (humidified)

Use tent or mask/nasal prongs. Do not use Ventimask.

Monitor O_2 levels in tent and maintain as high as possible. O_2 overdose for practical purposes is not a problem in childhood asthma.

2. Fluids
    Maintenance of hydration is very important. Give copious fluids orally or if i.v. allow for increased losses from respiration, but beware of possible pulmonary oedema in very severe asthma.

3. Alkali
    i.v. bicarbonate to raise pH to 7.3 if pH less than 7.1 (*see* p.1).

4. Antibiotics
    If clear evidence of secondary bacterial infection.
    Penicillin is antibiotic of first choice.

5. Sedation
    Sedatives are contraindicated – restlessness is usually due to hypoxia.

6. Physiotherapy
    Not useful in the very acute stage but should be started once child less dyspnoeic. Arrange for postural coughing 10-15 minutes after salbutamol inhalations.

Subsequent Management

1. Drug therapy
    If given steroids, continue i.v. 24-48 hours then stop or change to oral prednisone 2mg/kg 6-8 hourly. Reduce dosage rapidly over 48 hours depending on progress.
    As clinical improvement occurs, salbutamol inhalations may be reduced to p.r.n., at same time introducing oral bronchodilators (*see* Pharmacopoeia).
    Consider long term prophylaxis with sodium cromoglycate and/or betamethasone inhalations.

2. Assessing precipitating factors
    allergic
    psychological
    infective
    environmental, e.g. parents' smoking

3. Have parents instructed in techniques of postural coughing where onset seems to follow URTI. Some children/parents find breathing exercises helpful.

4. Respiratory function tests just prior to discharge provide useful information.

5. Start growth chart of height and weight.

BACTERIAL PNEUMONIA

Investigations
1. Microbiology – *see* Asthma (p.110)
2. Sputum, if possible, for culture and sensitivity
3. Blood screen
4. ESR
5. Blood culture
6. Chest X-ray – PA and lateral erect film (? fluid level in abscess)
7. Skin test for TB

Management
1. Oxygen
2. Sponge and fan to decrease temperature
3. Physiotherapy
4. Antibiotic therapy.
   The majority of cases are due to pneumococcus and will respond to penicillin. If an abscess is seen, consider staph.
5. If pleural involvement – consider drainage.

Staphylococcal Pneumonia

Penicillin 1-2 megaunits 4-6 hourly i.v.
Cloxacillin 200-400mg/kg/day. Four times a day i.v.
Ten days treatment
When sensitivities become available, stop unnecessary drug.

Str. Pneumoniae

Penicillin $\frac{1}{2}$-1 megaunit i.m. or i.v. stat. and then oral dose for age for 5 days.

Observations
1. Daily physical examination ? developmental of pleural effusion; empyema.
2. Watch for onset of sputum production. Generally indicates resolution.

3. If slow to clear, consider possibility of foreign body.
4. X-ray. Repeat at 48 hours and 7 days, or if signs of complications develop.
5. Blood screen and ESR. Repeat after 48 hours and 7 days.

ACUTE BRONCHIOLITIS IN INFANCY

Investigations

1. Microbiology – *see* Asthma (p.110)
2. Chest X-ray
3. Blood screen with differential w.b.c.
4. Urea and electrolytes
5. Capillary blood gases – as baseline on admission and to monitor progress as indicated.

Management

1. Maintain in high humidity
2. Oxygen:
   croupette/oxygen cot.
   nasal catheter if necessary
3. Rehydrate – i.v. if necessary (*see* p.49)
4. Frequent gentle suction and turning
5. Trial of salbutamol by inhalation is warranted but it is usually ineffective in this age group.

Complications

1. If no improvement after management as above, or deterioration as shown by blood gases, then some will give hydrocortisone hemisuccinate 4mg/kg 2 hourly i.v.
2. If rising $P\text{CO}_2$ consider need for ventilation
3. Observe closely for development of heart failure. If this occurs, digitalise.
   Note:
   Apparent increase in size of liver may be result of flattening of diaphragm and not heart failure *per se*.
4. Penicillin if evidence of secondary bacterial pneumonia. Modify antibiotic if necessary following culture reports..

CROUP

Note:

If child presents with 'croup', but is severely distressed DO NOT examine the throat, because if the child has haemophilus epiglottitis this may precipitate complete respiratory obstruction leading to death. In this situation treat as for haemophilus epiglottitis.

Investigations

1. Microbiology (*see* Asthma p.110)
2. Chest X-ray
3. Blood screen with differential w.b.c.
4. Capillary gases for pH and $P\text{CO}_2$

Management

1. No sedation.
2. Croupette with HUMIDIFIED oxygen.
3. i.v. fluids if child not drinking (p.49).
4. Penicillin only if evidence of secondary bacterial infection.
5. If child fails to improve, or shows deterioration clinically, some will give hydrocortisone hemisuccinate 4mg/kg 2 hourly i.v.
6. If serial blood gases show rising $P\text{CO}_2$ consider ventilation.

CRITERIA FOR DIAGNOSIS OF RESPIRATORY FAILURE IN INFANTS AND CHILDREN WITH ACUTE PULMONARY DISEASE

These criteria must be considered as guidelines and not as absolute indications for mechanical ventilation or other extraordinary therapy.

One physiological criterion and any three of the following clinical features suggest a diagnosis of acute respiratory failure.

Clinical

1. Decreased or absent inspiratory breath sounds.
2. Severe inspiratory retractions and use of accessory muscles.
3. Cyanosis in 40% ambient oxygen.
4. Depressed level of consciousness and response to pain.
5. Poor skeletal muscle tone.

Physiological

Pa_{CO_2} – more than 8.64-9.31kPa (65-70mm Hg) arterial blood
Pa_{O_2} – less than 13.3kPa (100mm Hg) in 100% oxygen

Pulmonary Function

Vital capacity	50-70ml/kg
Tidal volume	approx. 6ml/kg
Dead space	approx. 2ml/kg

HAEMOPHILUS EPIGLOTTITIS

If seen outside hospital, must be accompanied to hospital by a doctor who is prepared to pass an endotracheal tube or otherwise create an airway (*see* below).

Management

1. Notify consultant paediatrician and anaesthetist.
2. Posture – child in position of greatest comfort; usually sitting upright and leaning forward.
3. *Portable* chest X-ray if this investigation required.
4. Croupette with humidified oxygen and nasal catheter with humified oxygen if tolerated.
5. i.v. antibiotics:
   chloramphenicol 100mg/kg/day.
   (decrease after 24-48 hours to 75mg/kg/day)
   and/or
   ampicillin 200mg/kg/day according to the antibiotic sensitivity of local strains of *H. influenzae.*

6. Some also give i.v. hydrocortisone hemisuccinate 4 mg/kg/2 hourly.
7. No sedation – restlessness and distress often on basis of hypoxia.
8. Observe closely –
    clinically
    blood gases

If deteriorating (*see* p.116) or in severe respiratory difficulty on arrival, intubation or elective tracheostomy is necessary. Intubation should not be attempted by other than consultant anaesthetist except in an emergency situation.

In *extreme situation* where child is not able to achieve any air entry due to laryngeal oedema, attempt intubation, preferably with Portex tube (avoid if possible rubber cuffed tubes). If this proves impossible, insert three or four 14 gauge needles in the midline halfway between the thyroid cartilage and suprasternal notch. (*see* diagram below)

If child unable to achieve adequate air entry following this and anaesthetist is not available, then carry out laryngotomy (horizontal incision between thyroid and cricoid cartileges using knife or scissors). (*see* diagram below)

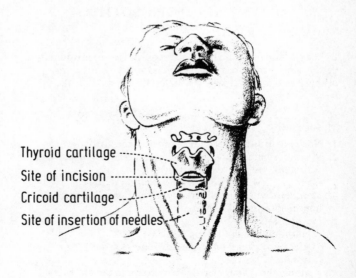

Thyroid cartilage ------
Site of incision ------------
Cricoid cartilage --------
Site of insertion of needles

Shock

Hypovolaemic Shock (*see* p.48)

Hypotension in Cardiac Failure (*see* pp. 9, 97)

Burns Shock (*see* p.2)

ENDOTOXIC SHOCK

Clinical Signs

Skin changes:
(a) Early – warm, dry
(b) Later – pale, damp, cold, cyanotic
Decreased blood pressure
Increased pulse rate
Increased respiratory rate but shallow
Decreased urinary output
Decreased awareness
Restlessness

Physiological changes in this form of shock may be divided
into an initial stage of peripheral vasodilation and a later stage
of peripheral vasoconstriction. Signs should be interpreted
with this in mind.

Immediate Investigations

1. Blood culture
2. Cross-match
3. Blood screen, differential, platelets
4. Urea and electrolytes
5. Blood gases

Immediate Management

1. Fluid replacement:
   0.9% saline or plasma 20ml/kg in 1 hour
2. Antibiotics:
   Ampicillin 400mg/kg/day in 6 divided doses i.v.
   Each dose run in over 20 mins.

Gentamicin 6mg/kg/day in 3 divided doses i.v.
Modify antibiotic according to blood culture results.
3. Hydrocortisone 50mg/kg i.v. stat.
Repeat hourly, if required, for 4 doses
Thereafter 15mg/kg 3 hourly up to 48 hours.

Monitor Therapy

1. Swan-Ganz catheter; if not available – CVP line
2. Blood pressure
3. Pulse rate
4. Respiratory rate
5. Urinary output

Further Management

1. i.v. infusion rate to be determined by central pressure. Use blood if Hb less than 100g/l.
2. Since by this stage the majority of patients will show signs of peripheral vasoconstriction use of isoprenaline should be considered.
   Withhold until central pressure is normal, then give isoprenaline 1mg/250ml 5% dextrose.
   Give 0.5-1ml/min under ECG control. Titrate against effect.
   Beware of ventricular arrhythmias.
   Stop if pulse rate more than 200/min.
3. Sodium bicarbonate. For dose *see* p.1).
4. O_2 by face mask.
5. If urine output low give a test dose of frusemide 2mg/kg stat. i.v.
   For normal urine output *see* p.5.

Further Investigations

1. CSF for sugar, protein, culture.
2. Skin swabs, urine for culture.
3. If disseminated intravascular coagulation suspected –
   Blood film, platelet count
   Thrombin clotting time
   Prothrombin clotting time, FDP
   PTTK, Factor assays
   Notify haematology consultant

Anaphylactoid Shock

1. Adrenaline 1:1000, 0.2-0.5ml s.c.
   Repeat in 5 min. if no response.
2. Chlorpheniramine maleate, 5-20mg i.m. stat.
3. Hydrocortisone – *see* Endotoxic Shock (p.119).
4. Fluids – *see* Endotoxic Shock (p.119).

Drug Index

Acetazolamide (Diamox)   29, 139
ACTH   151
Adrenaline   8, 97, 111, 121, 141
Alcobon (flucytosine)   137
Aldomet (methyldopa)   145
Alupent (Orciprenaline)   142
Aminophylline   7, 112, 141
Amitriptyline   149
Amoxil (amoxycillin)   32, 43, 44, 107, 132
Amoxycillin (Amoxil)   32, 43, 44, 107, 132
Amphotericin B (Fungilin, Fungizone)   137
Ampicillin   80, 81, 82, 117, 119, 132
Amylobarbitone Sodium (sodium amytal)   25, 139
Analgesics   131
Antibacterial   132
Antibiotics   19, 35, 39, 43, 54, 55, 84, 113, 114, 115, 117, 119, 132
Anticoagulants   139
Anticonvulsants   32, 139
Antidepressants   15, 91, 95
Anti-emetics   54
Antifungal   137
Antihistamines   45, 150
Anti-inflammatory agents   141
Antiparasitics   138
Antipyretics   141
Antispasmodics   130
Antiviral agents   138
Apresoline (hydrallazine)   100, 145
Aspirin   18, 91, 141
Atropine methonitrate (Eumydrin)   130
Atropine sulphate   146
Atrovent (ipratropium bromide)   142

Bactrim (co-trimoxazole)   107, 134
Beclomethasone dipropionate (Becotide)   141
Becotide (beclomethasone dipropionate)   141
Benadryl (diphenhydramine hydrochloride)   90
Benemid (probenecid)   136
Benzathine penicillin   19
Benztropine mesylate (Cogentin)   90
Benzyl penicillin   20, 86, 132
Betamethasone   43, 113

Gentamicin   84, 120, 135
Glucagon   97, 147
Glucocorticoids   147
Griseofulvin   137
Guanethidine (Ismelin)   144

Heparin   139
Human immunoglobulin (gamma globulin)   148
Hydrallazine (Apresoline)   100, 145
Hydrocortisone   120, 121
Hydrocortisone hemisuccinate   112, 118
Hydrocortisone sodium succinate   147
Hyperstat (diazoxide)   144
Hypotensive agents   144

Imipramine (Tofranil)   149
Inderal (propranolol)   143, 145
Insulin   37, 38, 39, 40, 41, 105
Intal (sodium cromoglycate)   113, 143
Ipratropium bromide (Atrovent)   142
Iron therapy   148
Ismelin   144
Isoniazid   135
Isoprenaline   8, 97

Kanamycin   135
Keflex (cephalexin)   133
Keflin (cephalothin)   133
Kefzol (cephazolin)   133

Largactil (chlorpromazine)   149
Lasix (frusemide)   7, 10, 97, 102, 144
Laxatives   130
Lignocaine   97, 143
Lincocin (lincomycin)   135
Lincomycin (Lincocin)   135

Mandelamine (methenamine mandelate)   135
Mannitol   83, 89, 149
Maxolon (metoclopramide)   150
Mebendazole (Vermox)   138
Melleril (thioridazine)   149
Merbentyl   130
Mestinon (pyridostigmine bromide)   146
Methanamine mandelate (Mandelamine)   135
Methicillin (Celbenin)   135
Methyldopa (Aldomet)   145
Methylphenidate (Ritalin)   149
Methyltestosterone   147

Pharmacopoeia

Note:

This handbook was originally prepared for use in New Zealand. Certain proprietary brands and certain formulations may be unavailable in some countries. In the following section, products unavailable in New Zealand at the time of going to press are marked thus * while products unavailable in the UK are marked thus †. Where doubt exists regarding preparations or dosages, consult MIMS or the manufacturer's literature.

ALIMENTARY SYSTEM

Antispasmodics

Atropine methonitrate (Eumydrin) 0.6%

> Solution – each drop (0.025ml) contains 0.15mg
> 0.3-0.6mg/kg/day in 5 divided doses given orally 20 mins before feed

Dicyclomine hydrochloride (Merbentyl)

> Syrup 10mg/5ml
> Less than 2 weeks 2.5-5mg 15 mins before feeds
> Infants 5-10mg 15 mins before feeds
> Maximum 4 doses in any 24 hours

Laxatives

Dioctyl sodium succinate (Dioctyl-Medo; † Coloxyl)

> Tab. 20mg
> ½-1 tab. 3 times daily
> Syrup 12.5mg in 5ml
> 5-10ml 2 or 3 times daily, or 5.15ml by enema

also Dioctyl-Forte

> Tab. 100mg
> 1 daily

Bisacodyl (Dulcolax)

>   Suppository 5mg, 10mg
>   \> 6yr. 1 × 5mg at night
>   Rectal solution 2.74mg/ml
>   1-2ml
>   Tab. 5mg
>   \> 6yr. 1 at night

Micralax

>   Liquid 5ml/micro-enema
>   1ml/yr. of age to 5ml max.

Senokot

>   Granules 15mg/5ml dose
>   ½-1 teaspoon as required
>   Tabs. 7.5 mg
>   1-2 tabs. as required

ANALGESICS
rarely required and poorly tolerated under age of 2 years

Narcotics

'Brompton Cocktail'

morphine hydrochloride	5mg
cocaine hydrochloride	5mg
alcohol 90%	0.625ml
syrup	1.25ml
chloroform water to	5ml

0.2ml/kg, i.e. = 0.2mg/kg/dose morphine. Increase as necessary

Codeine phosphate

>   Tab. 15mg, 30mg
>   3mg/kg/day in three divided doses
>   ***Note:** avoid in young children.*

Morphine sulphate

>   Injection 4, 8, 10, 15, 20 and 30mg/ml
>   0.2mg/kg/dose i.m. or s.c. Max. 15mg single dose

Pethidine

>   Tabs. 25mg, 50mg and 100mg
>   Injection 50mg/ml
>   1-2mg/kg/dose orally, i.m. or s.c.

Narcotic antagonists

Naloxone (Narcan/Neonatal Narcan)

> Solution 0.02mg/ml, 0.4mg/ml
> Neonates: 0.02mg/kg i.v., i.m. or s.c. Repeat at 2-3 minute intervals PRN
> Others: 0.01mg/kg i.v.

Non-narcotics

Paracetamol (Panadol) (as antipyretic *see* p.00)

> Elixir 120mg/5ml
> Tab. 500mg
> 25mg/kg/day in 4 divided doses

Pentazocine (Fortral)

> Injection 30mg/ml
> 1mg/kg i.m. or s.c.; 0.5mg/kg i.v. Repeat 4 times daily as necessary.
> Tab. 25mg, 50mg
> 5mg/kg/day in 3-5 divided doses

ANTIBIOTICS

Antibacterial

Amoxycillin (Amoxil)

> Syrup 125mg/5ml, 250mg/5ml
> Paediatric suspension 125mg/1.25ml; *tabs. 125mg
> Caps. 250mg, 500mg
> 125-250mg three times daily

Ampicillin

> Syrup 125mg/5ml, 250mg/5ml
> Paediatric suspension 125mg/1.25ml; *tabs. 125mg
> Caps. 250mg, 500mg
> Injection 100mg, 250mg, 500mg, 1g
> 50-100mg/kg/day orally, i.m. or i.v. in 4-6 divided doses
> In severe infections up to 400mg/kg/day i.v. may be given

Benzyl penicillin

> Injection vial = 1 mega unit = 600mg
> 25000-50000 units/kg/day in 4 divided doses i.m.
> In severe infections give 200 000-400 000 units/kg/day i.v.

Carbenicillin (Pyopen)

> Injection vials 1g, 5g
> 100-500mg/kg/day in 4 divided doses i.m. or i.v.
> By nebuliser: 1g 2-4 times daily

Cephalexin (Keflex)

> Suspension 125mg/5ml, 250mg/5ml
> Caps. 250mg, 500mg
> Tabs. 250mg, 500mg
> 25-100mg/kg/day in 4 divided doses
> Max. 4g/day

Cephazolin (Kefzol)

> Injection 500mg, 1g
> 25-100mg/kg/day in 3 or 4 divided doses i.m. or i.v.

Cephalothin (Keflin)

> Injection 1g
> 80-160 mg/kg/day in 4 divided doses i.m. or i.v.

Chloramphenicol

> Vial 1.2g
> Neonatal dose 25mg/kg/day i.v. in 4 divided doses
> 50-100mg/kg/day in 4 divided doses i.m. or i.v.
> Caps. 250mg
> Suspension 125mg/5ml

Clindamycin (Dalacin C)

> Syrup 75mg/5ml
> Caps. 75mg, 150mg
> 12-24mg/kg/day in 4 divided doses
> Injection 150mg/ml
> i.m. 10-30mg/kg/day
> i.v. 15-40mg/kg/day

Cloxacillin (Orbenin)

> Syrup 125mg/5ml
> Caps. 250mg, 500mg
> Injection 250mg, 500mg
> 50-100mg/kg/day in 4 divided doses

Colistin (Colomycin)

> * Injection vial 500 000 units, * 1 000 000 units
> 50 000 units/kg/day in 3 divided doses i.m. or i.v.
> † Injection vial 150mg (80mg of colistin sulphomethate =
> 1 000 000 units) 2-5mg/kg/d in 2 to 4 divided doses i.m.or
> i.v.

Co-trimoxazole (Bactrim, Septrin)

> Paediatric suspension and syrup:
>   40mg trimethoprim
>   200mg sulphamethoxazole, } 5ml
> Paediatric tabs.
>   20mg trimethoprim
>   100mg sulphamethoxazole
> i.e. 1 paediatric tab. = 2.5ml paediatric suspension

> **Note:** 1 adult tab. (80mg trimethoprim, 400mg
> sulphamethoxazole) = 4 paediatric tabs. = 10ml paediatric
> suspension or syrup
> Dose 0.5ml (or equiv.)/kg/day in 2 divided doses

> Infusion:
>   80mg trimethoprim,
>   400mg sulphamethoxazole } 5ml
> Dose 2ml/5kg/day in 2 divided doses
> i.m. ampoules:
>   160mg trimethoprim
>   800mg sulphamethoxazole } 3ml
> Dose 6-12yr. 1.5ml twice daily; > 12yr. 3ml twice daily

Erythromycin

> Suspensions 125mg/5ml, 250mg/5ml
> Paediatric drops 100mg/ml
> Tabs. 250mg, 500mg
> 30-50mg/kg/day in 4 divided doses

Ethambutol (Myambutol)

> Tabs. 100mg, 400mg
> 15mg/kg/day in a single daily dose

Flucloxacillin (Floxapen)

> Syrup 125mg/5ml
> Caps. 250mg
> Dose < 2yr 2.5ml 3 times daily; 2-10yr 5ml 3 times daily

Fusidic Acid (Fucidin)

> Suspension 250mg/5ml; Tab. 250mg 20-30mg/kg/day in 3
> divided doses with food
> Injection 500mg sodium fusidate/vial 20mg/kg/day in 3
> divided doses. Slow infusion

Gentamicin

> Injection 80mg/2ml, 20mg/2ml; 5mg/ml for intrathecal use
> neonates 6mg/kg/day in 2 divided doses i.m. or i.v.
> others 6mg/kg/day in 3 divided doses
> By nebuliser 20mg 2-4 times daily. Dilute to 2ml volume
> with 0.9% saline if necessary

Isoniazid

> Tabs. 50mg, 100mg
> 10-20mg/kg/day in 3 divided doses

Kanamycin

> Caps. 250mg
> 15-60mg/kg/day in 4 divided doses
> Injection 1g/3ml, 1g/4ml; † 0.25g/2ml
> 15mg/kg/day in 2 divided doses i.m.

Lincomycin (Lincocin)

> Syrup 250mg/5ml
> Caps. 500mg, † 250mg
> 30-60mg/kg/day in 4 divided doses
> Injection 300mg/ml
> 10-20mg/kg/day in 3 divided doses i.m. or i.v.

Methenamine mandelate (Mandelamine)

> Tabs. * 250mg, 500mg, † 1g
> 100mg/kg stat. 50mg/kg/day in 4 divided doses

Methicillin (Celbenin)

> Vial 1g
> 100-400mg/kg/day in 4 divided doses i.m.

Metronidazole (Flagyl) for anaerobic infections (*see* also p.138)

> Tabs. 200mg, 400mg
> Suppos. 500mg, 1g
> Infusion 500mg/100ml
> 20mg/kg/day in 3 divided doses (i.v. give each dose over
> 20 mins)

Nalidixic acid (Negram)

> Suspension * 60mg/ml, † 50mg/ml
> Tabs. 500mg
> 50mg/kg/day in 4 divided doses

Neomycin

> Tabs. 0.5g
> 50-100mg/kg/day in 4 divided doses

Nitrofurantoin

> Susp. 25mg/5ml
> Tabs. 50mg, 100mg
> Caps. † 50mg, † 100mg
> 5-10mg/kg/day in 4 divided doses with meals

Penicillin V

> Syrup and suspension 125mg/5ml, 250mg/5ml
> Tabs. and caps. 125mg, 250mg, † 500mg
> 50mg/kg/day in 4 divided doses

Polymyxin B

> Injection vial 500000 units = 50mg
> 1.5-2.5mg/kg/day in 4 divided doses i.m. or i.v.

Probenecid (Benemid)

> *Not an antibiotic, but is employed to elevate plasma level of
> certain antibiotics, notably the penicillins and
> cephalosporins (except cephaloridine).*
>
> Tabs. 500mg
> Stat dose 25mg/kg, then 40mg/kg/day in 4 divided doses.
> Give approx. 30 min before a penicillin or cephalosporin

Rifampicin

> Caps. 150mg, 300mg
> Tabs. † 450mg, † 600mg
> Syrup 100mg/5ml
> Up to 20mg/kg/day. Single pre-breakfast dose. Max daily
> dose 600mg

Streptomycin

> Vial 1g
> 30mg/kg/day in 2 divided doses i.m. Max dose 1g/day. In
> TB give as a single daily injection

Sulphadimidine

> Tabs. 500mg
> 150-200mg/kg/day in 4 divided doses
> Injection vial 1g/3ml
> 125mg/kg/day i.m. or i.v. in 4 divided doses

Ticarcillin disodium (* Ticar; † Tarcil)

> Injection vial 1g, 3g, * 5g
> 200-300mg/kg/day in divided doses every 4-6 hours by i.v.
> infusion

Tobramycin sulphate (Nebcin)

> Injection vial, * 10mg/ml, 40mg/ml
> 3-5mg/kg/day in 3 divided doses i.m. or slowly i.v.
> Neonates 3-4mg/kg/day in 2 divided doses
> By nebuliser 20mg 2-4 times daily – dilute to 2ml with
> 0.9% saline

Antifungal

Amphotericin B

> Suspension 100mg/ml (Fungilin)
> * Tabs. 100mg; lozenges 10mg (Fungilin)
> 1ml suspension or 1 lozenge held in mouth 4 times daily
> Injection vial 50mg (Fungizone)
> 0.25mg/kg/day by slow i.v. infusion in 5% dextrose
> (concentration 0.1mg/ml) over 6 hours. Slowly increase to
> max 1mg/kg/day

Flucytosine (Alcobon)

> Tabs. 500mg
> 100-200mg/kg/day in 4 divided doses
> Infusion 2.5g in 250ml
> 37.5-50mg/kg i.v. 6 hourly. Give over 20-40 minutes

Griseofulvin

> Suspension 125mg/5ml
> Tabs. 125mg, 500mg
> 10mg/kg once daily

Natamycin (Pimafucin)

> Suspension (oral) 1%
> Suspension (aerosol) 2.5%, † Tabs. 100mg
> Infant dose 1% suspension, 4 drops under tongue after
> every feed

Nystatin (Nystan)

> Suspension (oral) 100 000 units/ml
> 1ml 4 times daily, spread into recesses of mouth, for oral infection

Antiparasitic

Bephenium hydroxynaphthoate (Alcopar) *for hookworm, roundworm and whipworm*

> Granules 5g sachets
> 2.5-5g single dose

Mebendazole (Vermox) *broad spectrum*.

> Tab. 100mg
> Suspension 100mg/5 ml
> *For pinworm or threadworm* 100mg single dose, repeat one week later
> *Other worms* 100mg twice daily for 3 days

Metronidazole (Flagyl) *for Giardia lamblia (see* also p.135)

> Tabs. 200mg, 400mg
> 40mg/kg/day in one dose – three day course

Tinidazole (Fasigyn) *for Giardia lamblia*

> Tabs. 500mg
> 0.5-2g single dose

† Viprynium embonate (Vanquin) *for threadworm*

> Suspension 10mg/ml
> Tabs. 50mg
> 5mg/kg/stat. Repeat after one week. Treat whole family

Antiviral

Vidarabine monohydrate (Vira-A)

> Vial 1g, 200mg/ml
> *Chickenpox and disseminated Herpes zoster*
> 10mg/kg/day for 5 days
> *Herpes simplex encephalitis*
> 15mg/kg/day for 10 days. See manufacturer's literature for details of administration

ANTICOAGULANTS

Heparin

Injection vials 1000, 5000, 25 000 units/ml
Loading dose 150-200 units/kg i.v. as single dose
Maintenance 400-800 units/kg/day in continuous i.v.
infusion.
Aim for PTT × 2 normal

ANTICONVULSANTS

Acetazolamide (Diamox)

Caps. 500mg (Sustet – gradual release)
Tabs. 250mg
Injection 500mg
10-30mg/kg/day in 3 divided doses

Amylobarbitone sodium (Sodium amytal)

Tabs. 30mg, 60mg, 100mg, 200mg
Caps. 200mg
Injection amps. 250mg, 500mg (*see* p.26)

Carbamazepine (Tegretol)

Syrup 100mg/5ml
Tabs. * 100mg, 200mg, † 400mg
10-30mg/kg/day in 2-4 divided doses – introduce
gradually
Therapeutic Plasma Level (TPL) 6-12μg/ml

Clonazepam (Rivotril)

Tabs. 0.5mg, 2mg, † Oral drops 2.5mg/ml
Injection ampoules 1mg
0.1-0.2mg/kg/day in 2 divided doses
TPL = 0.025-0.075μg/ml
For status epilepticus give 0.5mg i.v. *slowly*

Diazepam (Valium)

Syrup 2mg/5ml
Caps. 2mg, 5mg
Tabs. 2mg, 5mg, 10mg, † Suppos. 5mg
0.1-1mg/kg/day in 3 divided doses
For status epilepticus give 0.25mg/kg *slowly i.v.* (*see* p.25)

Ethosuximide (Zarontin)

>Syrup 250mg/5ml
>Caps. 250mg
>15-50mg/kg/day in 2 divided doses
>TPL = 40-120μg/ml

Nitrazepam (Mogadon)

>Caps. 5mg
>Tabs. 5mg
>2.5mg nocte initially
>0.15-2mg/kg/day in 2 to 3 divided doses

Phenobarbitone

>Elixir 15mg/5ml
>Tabs. † 7.5mg, 15mg, 30mg, 60mg, 100mg, † 125mg
>3-10mg/kg/day in 1 or 2 divided doses
>Injection phenobarbitone sodium 200mg/ml (*see* p.26)
>TPL = 10-30μg/ml

Phenytoin (Epanutin)

>Suspension 30mg/5ml, † 100mg/5ml
>Caps. * 25mg, † 30mg, * 50mg, 100mg
>* Tabs. 50mg (chewable)
>Injection amps. 250mg/5ml
>3-8mg/kg/day in 2-4 divided doses
>TPL = 10-20μg/ml

Primidone (Mysoline)

>Suspension 250mg/5ml
>Tabs. 250mg
>10-30mg/kg/day in 2-4 divided doses
>TPL = 10-30μg/ml (as phenobarbitone)

Sodium valproate (Epilim)

>Tabs. 200mg, * 500mg (enteric-coated)
>Syrup 200mg/5ml
>0-3 years 20-30mg/kg/day in 3 divided doses
>3-15 years 400mg/day in 3 divided doses and increase as
>necessary
>TPL = 50-100μg/ml

Steroids (*see* p.151)

Sulthiame (Ospolot)

> Tabs. 50mg, 200mg
> * Suspension 50mg in 5 ml
> 10-15mg/kg/day in 3 divided doses. Introduce gradually

ANTI-INFLAMMATORY AGENTS

Aspirin (for rheumatoid arthritis, rheumatic fever)

> Tabs. plain 300mg; enteric coated 300mg, * 600mg; † 650mg, soluble 300mg
> Initially 100mg/kg/day in 6 divided doses. Aim for blood level 25-35mg/dl

Steroids (*see* p.151)

ANTIPYRETICS

Aspirin

> 10mg/kg/dose up to 4 hourly (*see* anti-inflammatory agents)
> Usually best avoided in children under 2 years

Paracetamol

> Elixir 120mg/5ml
> Tabs. 500mg
> 10mg/kg/dose up to 4 hourly

ASTHMA MEDICATIONS

Adrenaline

> 1:100 solution (*see* p.112)

Aminophylline

> Injection 250mg/10ml (*see* p.113)

Beclomethasone dipropionate inhaler (Becotide)

> Aerosol 50μg/puff
> 1-2 puffs twice daily
> Rotacaps 100 and 200μg
> 100μg 2 to 4 times daily

Choline theophyllinate (Choledyl)

>Syrup 62.5mg/5ml
>Tabs. 100mg, 200mg
>15-20mg/kg/day in 4 divided doses

Theophylline (Nuelin)

>Tabs. † 50mg, 125mg, † 200mg, 175mg (SA), 250mg (SA), † 500mg (SA)
>Liquid * 62.5mg/5ml, † 80mg/15ml
>12-20mg/kg/day in 4 divided doses (only twice daily for sustained release tablets)
>*Note: TPL for Theophylline group*
>10-20µg/ml

Ethylnoradrenaline (Bronkephrine)

>Injection 2mg/ml (*see* p.113)

Ipratropium bromide (Atrovent)

>Aerosol 20µg/puff
>1-2 puffs 3 times daily

Orciprenaline (Alupent)

>Syrup 10mg/5ml
>Tabs. 20mg
>2mg/kg/day in 3-4 divided doses
>Injection 0.5mg/ml
>Aerosol 0.75mg/puff
>1-2 puffs 3-4 times daily

Salbutamol (Ventolin)

>Syrup 2mg/5ml
>Tabs. 2mg, 4mg
>1-2mg 3 or 4 times daily according to age
>Spandets 8mg
>Aerosol 100µg/puff. Rotacaps 200µg and 400µg by Rotahaler
>Inhaler 1-2 inhalations 4 hourly as required
>Injection * 0.05mg/ml, 0.5mg/ml, 1mg/ml
>i.v. (*see* p.113)
>Respirator solution 5mg/ml
>Inhalations in hospital (*see* p.112)

Sodium cromoglycate (Intal)

> Spincap 20mg, initially 1 spincap 4-6 times daily.
> Maintenance dose may be lower
> Nebuliser soln, amp 20mg/2ml, initially 1 ampoule 4 times daily by nebuliser. Maintenance dose may be lower

CARDIOVASCULAR SYSTEM

Cardiac

Calcium chloride

> Injection 10%
> 0.2ml/kg i.v. or intracardiac. Repeat at 30-60 minute intervals as required (*see* p.9)

Digoxin

> Elixir 0.05mg/ml
> Tabs. 0.0625mg, * 0.125mg, 0.25mg
> Injection 0.05mg/2ml, 0.5mg/2ml
> *To digitalise:* 0.08mg/kg/24 hours orally, or
> 0.06mg/kg/24 hours i.m. or i.v.
> Give ½ stat – after 12 hours ¼ – after another 12 hours ¼
> Maintenance 0.01-0.02mg/kg/day in 2 divided doses and adjust if necessary
> TPL = 1-2.5μg/ml

Lignocaine

> Use 1% soln. *without* adrenaline (1% soln: 10mg/ml)
> 2-3mg/kg over 5-10 minutes i.v., or i.m.
> Continuous infusion 0.1% soln. in 5% dextrose at 30-50μg/kg/minute

Procainamide

> Tabs. 250mg, Oral 30-50mg/kg/day in 6 divided doses
> 'Durules' (sustained action) 500mg
> Injection 100mg/ml
> i.v. 2mg/kg/dose slowly
> i.m. 6mg/kg/dose 4-6 hourly

Propranolol (Inderal) (*see also* p.145)

> Tabs. 10mg, 40mg, * 80mg, 160mg
> Maintenance 1mg/kg/dose 3-4 times a day
> Injection 1mg/ml

For severe hypoxic spell 0.1mg/kg i.v. slowly to maximum of 5mg (*see* p.8)

Quinidine

Tabs. (sulphate) 200mg, 300mg, 20mg/kg/day in 4-6 doses
Caps. 250mg, 'Durules' 250mg (equivalent to 200mg quinidine sulphate; sustained action) 10mg/kg/day in 2-3 doses

Diuretics

Chlorothiazide (* Saluric, † Chlotride)

Tabs. 500mg
10-40mg/kg/day in 2 divided doses

Frusemide (Lasix)

Tabs. 20mg, 40mg, 500mg
Paediatric liquid 1mg/ml, † oral soln. 10mg/ml
Infusion 250mg/25ml
Injection 20mg/2ml, 50mg/5ml
Acute diuresis 2mg/kg *stat* i.m. or i.v.
Maintenance 1-3mg/kg/day in 2 divided doses early morning and noon

Potassium supplements

Effervescent potassium chloride tabs. * 6.7 or 12mmol potassium/tab. also † 8 or 14mmol potassium/tab.
1-2mmol/kg/day in 2 divided doses
1mmol = 75mg KCl

Hypotensive agents

Diazoxide (*Eudemine, † Hyperstat)

Injection 15mg/ml
In cases where need to drop blood pressure rapidly:
5mg/kg rapidly i.v.
May be given up to 4 times in 24 hours

Guanethidine (Ismelin)

Tab. 10mg, 25mg
Injection 10mg/ml
0.2 mg/kg in single daily dose
Can increase weekly to 1mg/kg/day

Hydrallazine (Apresoline)

> Tabs. 25mg, 50mg
> 1mg/kg/day in 2 divided doses. Increase gradually to
> max. 5mg/kg/day
> Injection 20mg powder for reconstituting
> 0.1-0.2mg/kg i.m. or i.v. (given with reserpine – *see* p.101)

Methyldopa (Aldomet)

Tabs. 125mg, 250mg, 500mg
10-50mg/kg/day in 4 divided doses

Phentolamine (Rogitine)

> Injection 10mg/ml
> 0.1mg/kg i.v.

Propranolol (Inderal) (*see also* p.143)

> Tabs. 10mg, 40mg, 80mg, 160mg
> 1 mg/kg/day in 4 divided doses
> Increase to max. 5mg/kg/day
> Injection 1mg/ml
> 0.01-0.1mg/kg/dose i.v. *slowly*

Reserpine (Serpasil)

> Injection 2.5mg/ml
> 0.01-0.07mg/kg *stat* i.m.
> ± hydrallazine 0.1-0.2mg/kg i.m.
> Repeat twice daily (*see* p.101)
> Tabs. 0.1mg, 0.25mg
> Oral maintenance 0.01-0.03mg/kg/day in 2 divided doses
> ± hydrallazine 1mg/kg/day. Increase if necessary to
> 5mg/kg/day

Sodium nitroprusside (Nipride)

> Injection 50mg vial
> Commence with $1\mu g/kg/min.$ i.v. and titrate against effect
> (maximum $8\mu g/kg/min.$)

CHOLINERGIC BLOCKERS

Atropine sulphate

Tab. * 0.5mg, † 0.6mg
Injection 0.4mg/ml, 0.6mg/ml
0.01mg/kg/dose oral, s.c. or i.m. (max. 0.4mg); repeat 2 hourly if necessary until adverse effects preclude further increase

CHOLINESTERASE INHIBITORS

Edrophonium chloride (Tensilon)

Injection 10mg/ml
Myasthenia gravis test: 0.2mg/kg. Give ⅕ slowly i.v. over 1 minute. If tolerated, give remainder.
Warning: *when testing, keep atropine sulphate syringe ready*

Neostigmine
Tabs. 15mg
2mg/kg/day 2-4 hourly
Injection 0.5mg/ml, 2.5mg/ml
Myasthenic crisis 0.04mg/kg i.m.

Pyridostigmine bromide (Mestinon)
Tab. 60mg
7mg/kg/day given in 4-6 divided doses
Injection 1mg/ml
In poisoning by tricyclic antidepressants 0.01mg/kg/dose i.v. every 1-4 hours

COUGH SUPPRESSANTS

Codeine linctus

15mg codeine/5ml
1-2mg/kg/day in 3-4 divided doses

ENDOCRINE

Adrenogenital syndrome

(a) salt losing crisis

1. i.v. fluids

0.9% saline in 10% dextrose 100ml/kg for first 24 hours.
(Plasma initially if shocked).

2. Glucocorticoids

Hydrocortisone sodium succinate

Injection 100mg/2ml
1-2mg/kg 4-6 hourly i.v.

3. Mineralocorticoids

* Deoxycortone acetate

Injection ampoule 5mg/ml
1-5mg i.m. daily

(b) maintenance treatment for salt losing type

1. Mineralocorticoids

Fludrocortisone 21-acetate (Florinef)
Tabs. 0.1mg, 1mg
0.05-0.2mg/day (check BP regularly)

2. Glucocorticoids (if necessary)

Cortisone acetate

Tabs. 5mg, 25mg
$24mg/m^2$/day in 3 divided doses

or

Prednisone

Tabs. 1mg, † 2.5mg, 5mg
0.14mg/kg/day in 2 divided doses

Other treatments

Glucagon (*see also* p.98)

Injection 1mg, 10mg
$50\mu g$/kg i.v. s.c. or i.m. every 30 minutes

Methyltestosterone

Tabs. 5mg, 10mg, 25mg, 50mg
1-2mg/kg/day

Thyroxine (Eltroxin)

Tabs. 0.05mg, 0.1mg
Under 1 year 0.025mg/day and increase
Over 1 year 0.0025-0.005mg/kg/day

Thyroid inhibitor

Carbimazole (Neo-Mercazole)

Tabs. 5mg
0.4mg/kg/day in 3 divided doses

Pancreatic enzyme supplements

Note: Stated doses are guidelines only. Considerably higher doses are sometimes necessary

Cotazym caps (Lipase, trypsin, amylase)

2-3 caps. with each meal

Cotazym B tablets (Lipase, trypsin, amylase, oxbile extract and cellulase)

1-2 tablets with each meal

Pancreatin BP granules (Pancrex)

5-15g dry or with water before meals

Pancrex V caps. and powder (5 times trypsin and lipase activity of Pancreatin BP)

Cap. 340mg 1-3 caps. – contents sprinkled on food
Powder 0.5-2g 4 times daily

† Viokase

Powder, caps. 305mg, tab. 325mg
3 tabs., 5 caps. or 0.75g powder ($\frac{1}{3}$ teaspoonful) with meals

GAMMA GLOBULIN (Human immunoglobulin)

Injection 160mg/ml i.m.
Prevention of infective hepatitis 0.02-0.04ml/kg
Rubella 0.6ml/kg (does not prevent viraemia)
Polio 0.3ml/kg
Measles 0.2ml/kg
Chicken pox in malignant diseases 5-7.9ml of ZIG (zoster immune globulin)

IRON THERAPY

(*see* haematology p.76)

PSYCHOTHERAPEUTIC DRUGS

Amitriptyline

    Syrup 10mg/5ml
    Tabs. 10mg, 25mg, 50mg
    Caps. 75mg
    For enuresis: 5-10 years, 10-20mg at night; over 10 years, 25-50mg at night
    Other uses 1mg/kg/day in 2 divided doses

Chlorpromazine (Largactil)

    Syrup 25mg/5ml
    Tabs. 10mg, 25mg, 50mg, 100mg
    Suspension 100mg/5ml
    Suppository 100mg
    Injection * 10mg/ml, 25mg/ml (i.m.)
    2mg/kg/day in 3 divided doses
    Note: Much higher doses occasionally used

Imipramine (Tofranil)

    Tabs. 10mg, 25mg
    * Syrup 25mg/5ml
    For enuresis: 4-10 years, 25mg at night; over 10 years, 50mg at night

Methylphenidate (Ritalin)

    Tab. 10mg
    Injection 20mg/2ml
    0.25-2mg/kg/day in 2 divided doses after breakfast and lunch
    Double initial dose weekly until effect obtained, side effects occur or max. dosage reached

Thioridazine (Melleril)

    Syrup 25mg/5ml, † oral soln. 30mg/ml
    Suspension * 25mg/5ml, † 50mg/5ml, * 100mg/5ml and † SR tab. 200mg
    Tabs. 10mg, 25mg, 50mg, 100mg
    1mg/kg/day in 3 divided doses

OSMOTIC INFUSIONS

Mannitol

    Injection 5%, 10%, 20%, 50ml ampoule, 500ml bottle

For cerebral oedema 0.25g/kg i.v. stat.
In oliguria or anuria, test dose of 0.2g/kg i.v. over 3-5
minutes should produce 6-10ml/kg urine in 1-3 hours

SEDATIVES AND ANTIHISTAMINES

Chloral hydrate

> Elixir paed. 200mg/5ml
> 30mg/kg/dose

Chlorpheniramine (Piriton)

> Syrup 2mg/5ml
> Tabs. (long acting) 8mg, * 12mg
> Tabs. 4mg
> Caps. (long acting) † 8mg, † 12mg
> Injection (s.c. or i.m.) ampoules 10mg/ml
> 0.35mg/kg/day in 3 divided doses

Pethidine co. injection contains

> chlorpromazine 6.25mg
> promethazine hydrochloride 6.25mg
> pethidine 25mg/ml of mixture
> 0.1 ml/kg i.m. Max. 1.5ml

Promethazine hydrochloride (Phenergan)

> Elixir 5mg/5ml
> Tabs. 10mg, 25mg
> 0.5-1mg/kg/day single dose
> Injection 25mg/ml
> 0.5mg/kg/day single dose i.m. or i.v.

Trimeprazine (Vallergan)

> Syrup 7.5mg/5ml
> Syrup forte 30mg/5ml
> Tabs. 10mg
> 2mg/kg/day
> Can use 2-4mg/kg as pre-anaesthetic medication

Sedation for jejunal biopsy

Quinalbarbitone sodium (Seconal) *and* Metoclopramide
(Maxolon)

Quinalbarbitone sodium (Seconal)	*and*	Metoclopramide (Maxolon)
Caps 50mg, 100mg		Paediatric liquid 1mg/ml
		Syrup 5mg/5ml
		Tabs. 10mg
		Injection 5mg/ml

Age (months)		
6-12	50-75mg	2-3mg
12-24	100mg	3-5mg
over 24	150mg	5-10mg

STEROIDS

Equivalent doses

cortisone	25mg
hydrocortisone	20mg
prednisone	5mg
prednisolone	5mg
methyl prednisolone	4mg
triamcinolone	4mg
paramethasone	2mg
betamethasone	0.7mg
dexamethasone	0.75mg

STEROID THERAPY IN SPECIAL CONDITIONS

Cerebral oedema

Dexamethasone

Tabs. 0.5mg, * 0.75mg
Injection vial 4mg/ml, † 5mg/ml
0.5-1mg/kg/ stat i.m. or i.v.
then
0.25-0.5mg/kg/day in 4 divided doses

Infantile spasms

ACTH

Injection vial 25 units/ml, 40 units/ml
40 units/day i.m. or s.c. initially

If synthetic preparation is used:
>   Tetracosactrin – amp. 0.25mg (Synacthen)
>   (1mg Tetracosactrin = 100 units ACTH)
>   Long acting ACTH gel 40 units/ml
>   80 units i.m. alternate days

Prednisone

>   Tabs. 1mg, † 2.5mg, 5mg
>   2-3mg/kg/day

For the following conditions see text

Subject Index